PHILOSOPHY

PHILOSOPHY OF MEDICINE an introduction

HENRIK R. WULFF MD
Consultant Physician, Department of Medical Gastroenterology
Herlev University Hospital, 2730 Herlev, Denmark

STIG ANDUR PEDERSEN
Professor of the Theory of Science
Roskilde University Centre, 4000 Roskilde, Denmark

RABEN ROSENBERG MD
Consultant Psychiatrist, Department of Psychiatry O
Rigshospitalet, 2100 Copenhagen, Denmark

INTRODUCTION BY
ANTHONY STORR FRCP, FRCPsych

SECOND EDITION

OXFORD
BLACKWELL SCIENTIFIC PUBLICATIONS
LONDON EDINBURGH BOSTON
MELBOURNE PARIS BERLIN VIENNA

©1986, 1990 by
Blackwell Scientific Publications
Editorial Offices:
Osney Mead, Oxford OX2 0EL
25 John Street, London WC1N 2BL
23 Ainslie Place, Edinburgh EH3 6AJ
3 Cambridge Center, Suite 208
  Cambridge, MA 02142, USA
54 University Street, Carlton
  Victoria 3053, Australia

All rights reserved. No part of this
publication may be reproduced, stored
in a retrieval system, or transmitted,
in any form or by any means,
electronic, mechanical, photocopying,
recording or otherwise without the prior
permission of
the copyright owner

First published 1986
Second edition 1990

Photoset by Enset (Photosetting),
Midsomer Norton, Bath, Avon
and printed and bound in
Great Britain

DISTRIBUTORS

Marston Book Services Ltd
PO Box 87
Oxford OX2 0DT
(*Orders:* Tel: 0865 791155
Fax: 0865 791927
Telex: 837515)

USA
Year Book Medical Publishers
200 North LaSalle Street
Chicago, Illinois 60601
(*Orders:* Tel: (312) 726-9733)

Canada
The C.V. Mosby Company
5240 Finch Avenue East
Scarborough, Ontario
(*Orders:* Tel: (416) 298-1588)

Australia
Blackwell Scientific Publications
(Australia) Pty Ltd
54 University Street
Carlton, Victoria 3053
(*Orders:* Tel: (03) 347-0300)

British Library
Cataloguing in Publication Data

Wulff, Henrik R.
  Philosophy of medicine: an
  introduction—2nd ed.
  1. Medicine—Philosophy
  I. Title II. Pedersen, Stig Andur
  III. Rosenberg, Raben
  610'.1 R723

ISBN 0-632-02948-X

CONTENTS

INTRODUCTION, viii

PREFACE, xiii

1 THE PARADIGM OF MEDICINE, 1
Kuhn's theory of science, 2
New trends in medical thinking, 7
Notes and references, 12

2 EMPIRICISM AND REALISM: A PHILOSOPHICAL PROBLEM, 13
The empiricist position, 16
Popper's solution, 22
The realist alternative, 25
Notes and references, 28

3 EMPIRICISM AND REALISM: TWO OPPOSING TRENDS IN MEDICAL THINKING, 30
Speculative realism, 30
Realism under empirical control, 32
Early empiricist trends, 33
Medical thinking today, 37
Notes and references, 45

4 THE MECHANICAL MODEL, 46
A dialogue between two philosophically minded clinicians, 46
The problem of normality, 47
The threshold problem, 50
The feeling of illness, 52
The telos of life, 55
A comment, 58
Notes and references, 59

vi Contents

5 **CAUSALITY IN MEDICINE**, 61
The logic of causation, 61
Five clinical cases, 66
Notes and references, 72

6 **THE DISEASE CLASSIFICATION: AN INDISPENSABLE TOOL**, 73
The history of the classification of diseases, 75
The status of a disease entity, 77
Diseases as demons or divine ideas, 81
Consequences of the Platonist view, 83
Notes and references, 88

7 **PROBABILITY AND BELIEF**, 89
Two concepts of probability, 89
Two clinical examples, 92
Textbook knowledge and clinical practice, 95
The probability of hypotheses, 97
Notes and references, 103

8 **THE NATURALISTIC APPROACH TO PSYCHIATRY**, 105
How does one recognize mental disease? 106
The empiricist view, 108
Mental disease as abnormal biological function, 111
Mental disease as inappropriate behaviour, 112
Mental disease as a social problem, 115
The eclectic view, 116
Notes and references, 118

9 **HERMENEUTICS: THE NATURE OF MAN IN A WIDER PERSPECTIVE**, 121
Anxiety as a fundamental state of mind, 124
Hermeneutics and natural science, 130
Notes and references, 134

10 **MEDICINE AND SOCIOLOGY**, 135
From classical epidemiology to empiricist social medicine, 136
Criticism of empiricist sociology, 141
Analytical hermeneutics, 143
German hermeneutic social theory, 146
Critical theory, 149
Notes and references, 154

11 **PSYCHOANALYSIS: NATURAL SCIENCE OR HERMENEUTICS?** 157
Freudian psychoanalysis, 157
Psychoanalysis as science, 160
Psychoanalysis as a hermeneutic discipline, 162
A balanced view, 166
Notes and references, 170

12 MEDICAL ETHICS AS A PHILOSOPHICAL DISCIPLINE, 172
'Good' and 'ought', 173
Ethics on three levels, 175
The origin of morality, 176
The structure of ethical reasoning, 179
The wide reflective equilibrium, 184
Notes and references, 186

13 THE ETHICAL DIMENSION OF MEDICAL DECISIONS, 187
Problems on a ward round, 187
Autonomy and paternalism, 192
The ultimate decision, 197
Ethics and clinical research, 199
Notes and references, 202

14 THE MIND AND THE BODY, 203
Logical behaviourism, 208
The causal theory of the mind, 209
The identity theory, 211
Functionalism, 212
Interactionistic dualism, 214
A recapitulation, 216
Notes and references, 217

NAME INDEX, 219

SUBJECT INDEX, 221

INTRODUCTION

The philosophy of medicine is not a subject to which much attention is paid in British medical schools. Medical students, during their long professional training, are required to assimilate and retain an ever-increasing number of facts about an extraordinary variety of diseases. Their time is more than fully occupied in acquiring enough knowledge to satisfy their examiners; and most accept the way that medicine is currently practised without questioning the basic assumptions upon which that practice is based. When students become qualified doctors, the majority will lead extremely busy lives in which practical problems of diagnosis and treatment will leave little time for reflection. Even if they go into research rather than into clinical work, it is probable that their pursuit of knowledge will be governed by existing paradigms. In Western countries, scientific medicine, during this century, has been immensely successful. The majority of infections have been conquered by a combination of immunization and antibiotics. Diseases which used to be fatal, like pernicious anaemia and diabetes, have become readily treatable. Infant mortality has been greatly reduced, and the hazards of childbirth diminished. Yet much remains to be done. Genetic engineering holds out the promise that many genetic defects can be prevented or modified. There are still crippling, chronic diseases, like multiple sclerosis and rheumatoid arthritis, which can be neither prevented nor effectively treated. The mysteries of the body's own protective immune system have yet to be fully unravelled. It is certain that the next fifty years will bring forth as many exciting scientific advances as the past fifty years have done. With so much to do, and so much evidence to show that current methods of investigation are fruitful, it might be argued that preoccupation with the philosophy of medicine is otiose. One of the virtues of this challenging, clearly argued book is that it persuades one that the opposite is true. The authors, a philosopher, a psychiatrist and a gastroenterologist, believe that medicine has entered a new phase in which basic assumptions have to be questioned. Following Thomas Kuhn, author of *The Structure of Scientific Revolutions*, the authors affirm that medicine has now entered upon a period of 'paradigmatic instability'. That is, it is a period in which doctors need to look at what they are doing afresh, and to reconsider their roles and responsibilities toward their patients and society.

In a clear discussion of the philosophical differences between empiricism and realism, which is aimed at those who know nothing of philosophy, the authors point out that science and medicine have been dominated by the empiricist point of view. This, roughly speaking, is the philosophical school of thought taking origin from Locke, Berkeley and Hume, and culminating in logical positivism. Philosophers of this type are principally concerned with observable facts, and eschew moral or metaphysical speculation. Applied to medicine, this philosophical stance has had the valuable consequences of making doctors much more objective in assessing the results of treatment, and in comparing the efficacy of one treatment with another. The authors remind us that the strictly objective, 'scientific' approach to medical problems is comparatively new. Double-blind trials, the proper use of statistics and the like, are recent and welcome developments. But the empiricist stance has also led to the simplistic notion that health and disease can be easily defined and distinguished from each other; that diseases are entities which, as it were, attack patients from outside themselves; and that, if adequate resources were provided by the welfare state, the amount of disease within a given population could be greatly reduced.

In fact, a kind of Parkinson's law seems to have been established, which might be stated as follows. 'The more medical facilities which are provided, the more diseases are disclosed which demand treatment.' In both Denmark and Great Britain, the health services have come to cost more and more in real terms. Consultations and hospital admissions have risen; but waiting lists have not been eliminated. Indeed, for some operations, like hip replacement, they are so long as to be ludicrous. It is true that technical advances have made it possible to keep hopelessly ill people alive on life-support machines; that renal dialysis prolongs the lives of some sufferers from kidney disease; and that transplant surgery has given some victims of heart disease a few extra years of life. But all these advances have brought ethical problems in their train, and the effect upon the average expected life-span of the general population has been very small.

The idea that one can get reduced 'disease' by expanding the health services has proved illusory, and should perhaps lead to a new way of looking at what constitutes 'disease'. In a powerfully argued disputation between two imaginary clinicians, the authors point out that the concept of disease as merely biological dysfunction is quite inadequate. For different patients, the same 'disease', like a duodenal ulcer, may have quite different meanings. For one patient, all that the diagnosis implied was that he needed to have a short period of drug treatment in which he had every confidence. For another, not previously affected, the diagnosis caused fear for his life. A third patient was anxious that, if his employers discovered what was wrong with him, they might deny him promotion.

Moreover, what is registered by the observer as biological dysfunction depends upon his own preconceptions. There is no such thing as a purely objective observation. The authors conclude that the biological concept of disease must be superseded, or at least expanded, by a point of view which can take into account morals, values and meanings as well as 'objective' facts.

The notion that the causes of a particular disease are nearly always multiple is generally accepted by doctors; but the purely biological approach to medicine often means that subjective 'causes' are somewhat neglected. Thus, because pneumococci are regarded as the principal 'cause' of pneumonia, eliminating them with antibiotics may be thought sufficient treatment, without much attention being paid to why this particular individual became susceptible to infection at a particular time. The authors make clear distinctions between 'necessary' and 'sufficient' causes, and also between 'redundant' and 'non-redundant' factors. Interaction between social, personal, genetic and other factors in the causation of disease is far more complex than is generally realized. The authors point out that, when doctors treat a particular disease, they are usually able to pin-point a few non-redundant factors in the causal network, but remain quite ignorant of many contributory factors which ought also to engage their attention.

Moreover, what constitutes 'disease' is by no means always obvious. This is especially true in psychiatry, in which definitions of 'disease' are often changed. Is homosexuality to be regarded as a normal variant, a mental disorder, or a sign of moral degeneration? All three points of view have had their advocates within living memory. Is symptom-free hypertension, discovered during routine examination, to be reckoned as a disease or not? Discussion of these problems in philosophical terms quite properly undermines the simplistic view that diseases are easily definable entities which from time to time 'attack' people.

The authors persuade us that the empiricist notion of disease as clearly definable, biological dysfunction is manifestly inadequate, and fails to do justice to what the authors call 'the true constituent features of human nature'. Has any other philosophical approach anything to offer? The authors believe so, and examine and expound the ideas of the continental philosophers, Kierkegaard, Heidegger, Gadamer, Sartre and Habermas. These philosophers are far removed from empiricism, and deal in the groups of ideas summarized under the headings of phenomenology, existentialism, and hermeneutics. It becomes increasingly clear that what one regards as 'disease' or 'treatment' depends on one's view of the nature of man. If, for example, a doctor believes that *angst* is an inescapable part of the human condition, he will not immediately prescribe a tranquillizing drug when consulted by an anxious patient. A hermeneutic enquiry seeks to establish the meaning of phenomena and to interpret their significance. Because man is reflective, self-conscious, and capable of choice, he cannot, when ill, be regarded in the same light as a machine which has gone wrong. Anxiety and depression are not simply unpleasant symptoms which the doctor should abolish, but may be indicators pointing toward an individual's need to examine and modify his whole attitude to life.

In the same way, the hermeneutic approach to society is not

content merely to record the statistical relation between defined social variables. The authors tell us that methods have been developed by which motives, values and attitudes in societies can also be studied. Human social interaction cannot be comprehended unless these underlying concepts are also examined.

Modern medicine has confronted doctors with a wide range of ethical problems which their predecessors did not have to face. There is, at present, a good deal of discussion of such problems, as witnessed by the debate on the ethics of experimentation on human embryos. Questions of patient participation in drug trials, of 'informed consent', and of how much patients should be told about their illnesses are all matters demanding some kind of ethical guidelines which are ably discussed by the joint authors.

This book bears witness to the fruitfulness of an unusual collaboration. I do not know of any other book written jointly by a philosopher, a physician and a psychiatrist. Any doctor who reads it will, I think, feel that he has gained new insights and a new way of looking at his professional activities. I am sure that the authors are right in thinking that medicine is passing through a phase of 'paradigmatic instability'. Not long ago, a lawyer claimed to have 'unmasked' medicine in his series of Reith lectures which, to my mind, were intemperate and sometimes ill-informed. But, however wrong Ian Kennedy was in detail, the fact that he chose this subject attests the fact that the public are increasingly concerned to understand what doctors are doing, and less inclined to accept on trust what doctors do. The medical profession itself has, I think, been too complacent, and unduly reluctant to examine its own presuppositions. No one who reads and assimilates the contents of this book will any longer be content with a purely empirical, pragmatic approach to medical practice. As medicine advances, more and more questions will arise about preservation of life at all costs, so-called 'quality of life', and equitable distribution of scarce and costly forms of medical and surgical treatment. Doctors can no longer be content to get on with the job of saving life and easing pain without considering any deeper implications of what they are doing. *Philosophy of Medicine* is modestly called 'An Introduction' by its authors; but it is an introduction to a debate about values in medicine which has far-reaching implications and which will continue for many years to come.

Anthony Storr

PREFACE

During the preparation of this book, we have had those readers in mind who know something about medicine but nothing about philosophy, and we have tried to explain ourselves as simply as possible. Primarily, the book has been written for members of the medical profession, medical students and others employed in the health service; it is written for those who like caring for their patients and appreciate the importance of technological advances, but are worried that we shall forget that our patients are self-reflecting human beings and not just biological machines. The greater part of the book is devoted to an analysis of medical science, but we shall argue in several chapters that scientific medicine is no more than a tool, albeit a very important one, which serves a humanistic purpose.

It cannot be concealed that some of the topics which we shall discuss are complicated ones. The book is a mixture of easy and difficult chapters, of easy and difficult passages; and we invite the uninitiated reader to read slowly and, whenever necessary, to re-read the difficult parts until he feels that he understands the arguments. Quick reading may give the reader an impression of the contents of medical philosophy, but he will only draw the full benefits from his study if he engages himself in a dialogue with the text and tries to make up his mind whether he agrees or disagrees with the different points of view. (It will be noted that 'he' in this book is often used in the sense 'she or he'.)

The reader may sometimes feel that we are losing ourselves in subtle philosophical arguments. At the beginning of Chapter 2, for instance, we shall discuss whether or not a cow in the meadow really exists, and it may pass through the reader's mind that life is too short for contemplating this type of philosophical problem. We hope, however, that he will find out later that the discussion was not superfluous. We should have liked to write the book by starting with the presentation of everyday medical problems, which were then analysed and discussed in philosophical terms, but we found that it was sometimes easier to introduce the necessary theoretical concepts in a purely philosophical chapter and to apply these philosophical ideas to medical problems in the succeeding ones. Therefore, there are three chapters (2, 9 and 11) which are purely philosophical.

Philosophical theories, attitudes and traditions are often denoted by unfamiliar words, and the reader may feel that the number of *-isms* is confusing. Perhaps we could have omitted some of these terms, but we decided that it was one of the purposes of the book to teach the reader correct philosophical terminology. The book is an introduction to the philosophy of medicine, and it would not serve this end unless it introduced the reader to that terminology which is needed to understand more sophisticated texts. Should the reader forget the meaning of some of the words, the subject index will be found to show where the words were first defined or explained.

We also hope that the book will prove useful for readers outside the medical profession whose primary interest is that of philosophy. Medicine is at the same time a science, a technology and an art, and many important issues of contemporary philosophy are well illustrated by medical examples. Medical terms are used freely in the book, but we do not think that it will be difficult for the academically trained, non-medical reader to grasp the meaning of the medical problems, even though some of the words may be unfamiliar.

This book is the united effort of three authors—a philosopher, a psychiatrist and a medical gastroenterologist—and the preparation of the manuscript is the result of an arduous process lasting for more than two years, during which we met at regular intervals, exchanging drafts and discussing the different topics. We agreed from the beginning that we had to continue until we found that each chapter was both philosophically acceptable and medically relevant, and we are, all three of us, co-responsible for all parts of the book.

We are indebted to a number of people for their help. Mr Per Saugman of Blackwell Scientific Publications heard about the project at its earliest stage and immediately suggested that the book should be published in English. Many of our colleagues have offered valuable comments, and Marion R. Wulff, MB, BS, helped us with the preparation of the English text.

We also wish to thank Mrs Lise Nielsen and Mrs Jane Holm Nielsen who typed many of the drafts as well as the final version.

Henrik R. Wulff
Stig Andur Pedersen
Raben Rosenberg

CHAPTER 1
THE PARADIGM OF MEDICINE

A doctor who wishes to make himself unpopular in conversations with colleagues need only ask questions of the following kind:
- You think that it is healthy to bicycle to work in the morning. What exactly do you mean by health?
- You say that duodenal ulcers are psychosomatic. Do you believe that the body and mind are separate entities and that the thing called mind may cause changes in the body?
- You say that this therapy is unscientific. Which are your criteria for accepting a treatment as scientific?
- You do not think that alcoholism is a disease. What do you understand by a disease?

It is, of course, quite justified that questions like these are met with at least mild irritation. The doctors are discussing specific medical topics, and each time the inquisitive colleague confuses the issue by asking questions of a general nature. Doctors who are discussing medical topics have to use words like health and disease, and they would never succeed in reaching a conclusion if they did not presuppose a mutual consensus as regards the meaning of a large number of fundamental concepts. By asking these seemingly innocent but almost unanswerable questions, the inquisitive doctor contests this consensus, and he hints that his colleagues do not really know what they are talking about.

However, members of the medical profession need not be ashamed that they have not thought seriously about the basic concepts of medical science, because, according to the contemporary American physicist, Thomas S. Kuhn, the same can be said of the practitioners of all other scientific disciplines. Kuhn's book *The Structure of Scientific Revolutions* [1] plays an important role in the current debate among philosophers of science, and in this chapter some of his ideas will be briefly explained.

Kuhn's theory of science

Kuhn has introduced the important concept which he calls the *paradigm* of a science. It is very difficult to give a concise definition of this word, but briefly it is used as a collective term, encompassing all that which the practitioners of a particular scientific discipline take for granted. The paradigm constitutes the framework within which the scientists reason when they try to solve their scientific problems; it represents the premises of scientific thinking and, therefore, it is not usually considered a scientific problem in itself.

This explanation may seem rather vague and it will be easier to understand the importance of this concept when we add that the paradigm of a science has such components as the meaning of the most fundamental scientific concepts (e.g. health and disease in medicine), the boundary of the legitimate area of research (e.g. the boundary between those problems which are regarded as medical and those which are said to be the concern of other sciences), the basic theories (e.g. the mechanical model of disease which will be discussed in Chapter 4), the accepted methods of research, and the values to which the scientists commit themselves.

The components of the paradigm constitute what has been called the *tacit* knowledge of the scientific community [2]; it is never taught explicitly, but it is embedded in the contents of both textbooks and medical journals.

Kuhn also uses the word *paradigm* in a somewhat narrower sense, as the paradigms of a science are also those previously published reports of scientific investigations which serve as models for further research. In Kuhn's book scientific papers are sometimes called puzzle-solutions (solutions of scientific puzzles), and he uses this expression in the following passage, in which he summarizes what is meant by a paradigm:

> On the one hand, it stands for the entire constellation of
> beliefs, techniques, and so on shared by the members of a given

community. On the other, it denotes one sort of element in that constellation, the concrete puzzle-solutions, which employed as models or examples, can replace specific rules as a basis for the solution of the remaining puzzles of a normal science [3].

Most laymen probably expect that medical students are taught what is meant by, for instance, a state of health and a state of illness, and that they study in great detail the structure of the official disease classification, but, as all doctors know, this is not the case. As Kuhn points out, it is a general rule that 'scientists... never learn concepts, laws and theories in the abstract... ' [4]. Instead, they gradually learn to use these intellectual tools by reading their textbooks and by listening to lectures. Students and young doctors gradually learn to think as their teachers, and in the end, when they partake in the tacit knowledge of the profession, they feel at home in the academic milieu and are accepted as colleagues.

As a consequence of this teaching process, scientists may learn to 'talk easily and well about the particular individual hypotheses that underlie a concrete piece of current research', but in spite of that 'they are little better than laymen at characterizing the established basis of their field' [5]. This deficiency will remain unnoticed when medical scientists report the results of their research, but it is often revealed when they try to explain their research to the uninitiated. They may translate all the scientific terms into ordinary language and explain all the facts in great detail, but they may still take so many things for granted that they are not fully understood.

Medicine is not only a scientific, but also a practical discipline, and Kuhn's ideas are also applicable to clinical medicine. The specialist who lives for his work and spends most of his time in the company of colleagues may find it difficult to converse with people who have not been indoctrinated in the same way. He may, for instance, feel that he has given one of his patients an excellent account of the results of all the investigations, the resulting diagnosis and the cause of the symptoms, but it is quite possible that the patient, taking only a small interest in all this technical talk, will ask the following question: 'I understood perfectly well, Doctor, that my stomach produces too much hydrochloric acid, and that this acid has produced an ulceration in something which is called the duodenum, but why did I develop the pain this spring and how do I prevent it from happening again?' Patients have not, like doctors, been indoctrinated with the idea that a disease is a mechanical fault of the body and that everything is explained satisfactorily when this fault has been diagnosed. They want to hear something about those factors in their daily lives which caused their illness, but they do not always appreciate that our knowledge of the environmental determinants of most non-infectious diseases is extremely limited. Most medical scientists are happy to explore in as much detail as possible the workings of the human body and care little about the interaction with the environment.

It might easily be inferred from this discussion that Kuhn encourages scientists to analyse, as thoroughly as possible, the paradigm of their discipline, but he does nothing of the kind. On the contrary, he believes that it would be impossible to reach consensus, and that the attempt to do so would result in no more than 'continual and deep frustration' [6]. To explain this point he quotes Ludwig Wittgenstein, who discusses such common words as *a chair* and *a leaf* [7]. We learn to use these words at an early age as we acquaint ourselves with those attributes which are shared by some chairs and some leaves, but anybody who tries to formulate exact definitions that are acceptable to everybody is bound to fail. Chairs and leaves must be regarded as 'families of objects', which are constituted by a network of resemblances, and there is no single set of attributes which identifies all chairs and all leaves and excludes all other objects. The ability to recognize such networks and to identify such commonplace objects is part of everybody's tacit knowledge, and usually the lack of explicit definitions causes no problems in everyday conversation. Everybody understands what we mean when we refer to a chair or a leaf. In a similar way, scientists may not be able to define in exact terms the components of the paradigm which governs their activities, but that does not necessarily mean that the words which they use and the rules which they follow are unduly imprecise and that they do not serve their practical purpose sufficiently well.

As we shall explain later, we are not quite as diffident as Kuhn as regards the ability of scientists to analyse the framework of their reasoning, but we shall make no naive attempt to define basic concepts in exact terms. Inquisitive doctors who ask what is meant by words like health, disease, scientific or psychosomatic may provoke extremely useful discussions, if they ask their questions at

The Paradigm of Medicine 5

the right moment, but they should always remember that they, themselves, are unable to define what is meant even by a chair or a leaf.

Kuhn's particular interest is the history of science, and it is his thesis that scientific disciplines do not develop gradually but by leaps and bounds. For long periods of time the paradigm of a science remains unchanged and the scientists are busy solving their problems within the conceptual framework of that paradigm. However, such periods, which according to Kuhn's terminology represent *normal* science, do not last forever. Sooner or later a crisis sets in, the paradigm breaks down and a *scientific revolution* ensues. The unity of the scientific community is disrupted by the emergence of competing schools of thought, but after a while a new paradigm attracts the allegiance of more and more scientists and a new period of productive normal science follows.

As mentioned already, Kuhn does not believe that philosophical debate within the scientific community is altogether desirable. On the contrary, he claims that it is the strength of normal science that scientists simply accept the established paradigm and devote themselves to their research. Normal scientific activity constantly discloses new interesting problems which attract attention, and a productive paradigm may keep generations of scientists busy. At the same time the paradigm sets limits to the scientific activity, as the scientists will only attempt to tackle those problems which, in principle, can be solved within that particular framework of ideas. As mentioned above, Kuhn uses the expression that normal scientists are engaged in *puzzle-solving* activity; they solve their puzzles according to accepted rules.

From time to time the scientists produce results which conflict with established theories, and scientific problems arise which cannot be solved within the framework of the paradigm, but such *anomalies* do not at once lead to a paradigmatic change. The controversial results and the insoluble problems will simply, for the time being, be shelved, as the scientific community will not accept that there is something wrong with the paradigm. As Kuhn puts it, 'it is a bad carpenter who blames his tools' [8]. When, however, the anomalies accumulate, the paradigm gradually weakens, and that which was taken for granted is suddenly seen as a scientific problem in its own right. The scientists experience a feeling of professional insecurity and they may even engage themselves in philosophical discussions. The crisis has set in.

Kuhn, who is a physicist, is particularly interested in sciences like physics, chemistry and astronomy, and he illustrates his ideas with examples, like the Copernican revolution in the 16th century and the replacement of Newtonian physics by Einstein's relativity theory in this century. He writes that the examples of scientific revolutions can be 'multiplied *ad nauseam*', and it is quite true that it is easy to add to the list. For instance, the publication of Darwin's book *On the Origin of Species* in 1859 heralded a true Kuhnian revolution, which changed biology and caused repercussions throughout the academic world. Previously, all biological thinking had been firmly based on the doctrine of the immutability of animal species (*nulla species nova*), and the theory of evolution represented a completely new paradigm which influenced not only biologists, but also theologians and political philosophers. The history of medicine, which is as long as that of any other science, also offers many examples of paradigmatic shifts. At the beginning of the 19th century, for instance, doctors began for the first time to identify diseases with anatomical lesions and a completely new disease classification was established. Those who have attempted to read old medical texts will know that they are sometimes very difficult to understand; the words may be intelligible, but their medical meaning may be incomprehensible to us, if it was part of a paradigm which was abandoned centuries ago.

There can be no doubt that Kuhn is right when he claims that scientific revolutions take place and that normal science exists, but it does not follow from the examples that sciences always develop in conceptual leaps and bounds. As we shall explain later, Kuhn's theories are not accepted by everybody, and it cannot be excluded that the paradigm of a science may also develop gradually and that scientists, rather than being mere puzzle-solvers, may play an active role in this development.

It is particularly uncertain to what extent Kuhn's theory correctly describes the development of medicine, which differs in at least two ways from pure sciences like physics and chemistry. Firstly, medical doctors do not only concern themselves with basic research, but also with clinical research and the practice of medicine. This means that they cover the whole spectrum of activities which in other fields are often labelled science, technology and techniques. Secondly, medicine comprises a variety of subdisciplines, and it is too much to expect that all medical thinking is founded on a single paradigm and that an anatomist, a physician, a health inspector and a psychiatrist reason in exactly the same way.

In spite of these reservations, Kuhn's ideas are well suited as an introduction to the study of medical philosophy. Medical thinking may be based on a complex of related subdisciplinary paradigms, rather than on a single one, but the idea of a paradigm pertains no less to medicine than to other sciences, and the philosopher of medicine sees it as one of his main tasks to explore this element of tacit knowledge. Further, the paradigmatic basis of such an important area as clinical practice seems to be much less settled today than it was only a few decades ago, and although we shall not predict a Kuhnian revolution, it is justified to say that clinical medicine has entered a period of paradigmatic instability. We shall now briefly discuss this development and, at the same time, introduce some of the subsequent chapters.

New trends in medical thinking

Medicine as we know it today originated in the last century, when medical scientists began to investigate systematically the structure and function of the human organism in health and disease. The break with previous traditions caused considerable paradigmatic unrest, which even led to philosophical discussions in medical journals, but towards the end of the century it was generally accepted by the medical profession that medicine was a branch of natural science and that disease processes must be explained in anatomical and physiological terms. The so-called mechanical model of disease which we shall discuss in detail in Chapters 3 and 4 became an important component of the paradigm of clinical thinking, and clinical medicine at that time entered a stable productive phase which in Kuhn's terminology may well be called a period of normal science. Since then, medical scientists have been extremely busy 'solving their puzzles', and their solutions have had astonishing practical consequences. We need only mention milestones like the introduction of effective treatment of diabetes and pernicious anaemia, the development of modern anaesthesiology and the discovery of antibiotics. Most people within and without the medical profession were deeply impressed by these and numerous other scientific conquests, and it is not surprising that few doctors were interested in philosophical problems. As a typical example, the time-honoured course in philosophy, which for centuries had been obligatory for medical and all other students at the University of Copenhagen, was abolished in 1971. It was considered a complete waste of time.

This productive period of normal science still persists, in so far as medical science with its emphasis on laboratory research continues to produce important results, but during the last few decades the paradigm which was established a century ago has been attacked from different angles.

In the 1960s, an increasing number of clinicians began to question the efficacy of all the new drugs which in those years gained access to clinical practice. Until then, it had been assumed that the clinical effect of new drugs could be predicted from laboratory studies of their mechanism of action, but now sceptical clinicians demanded direct empirical proof of their efficacy in the form of carefully controlled clinical trials. These clinicians, who established what may now be called the *critical clinical school*, took a great interest in research methods and biostatistics, and the double-blind randomized therapeutic trial was seen as the ideal—or paradigm—of clinical research. In Chapter 2 we shall discuss the historical and philosophical background of this development which may be seen as the culmination of an age-old tension between realism and empiricism in medical science.

A few years later—in the late '60s and the early '70s—clinicians in different parts of the world developed an interest in medical ethics. This new development was not, as might be imagined, a reaction to the strict scientific attitude which characterized the supporters of the critical clinical school, but represented a natural consequence of that attitude. Some of the first clinicians to take an interest in the ethics of medicine were themselves advocates of clinical research, who realized that their demand for controlled clinical trials created ethical problems which had to be analysed; and the combined interest in medical research and medical ethics led to the adoption of the Helsinki Declaration by the World Medical Association in 1964 (see p. 200). The interest in clinical

The Paradigm of Medicine 9

research and the interest in medical ethics were both prompted by a wish to curb the uninhibited introduction of new medical techniques into clinical practice. Controlled clinical studies serve to prevent the introduction of new preventive, diagnostic or therapeutic methods, if they are no better, i.e. no more effective, than those already in current use, whereas ethical reasoning helps us to decide whether the effects of new techniques are good in themselves, i.e. morally acceptable. Ethical questions were of less importance in those days when doctors could do little for their patients, but they could no longer be ignored when it became possible to transfer vital organs from one person to another, to diagnose congenital abnormalities in the fetus and to prolong the life of hopelessly ill patients. The medical profession had at long last learnt to appreciate that clinical practice is not only applied natural science, but that clinical decisions always include value judgments. As a result of this realization contemporary clinicians do not only talk about cures and survival, but also about their patients' quality of life. We shall return to this important topic in Chapter 12.

Psychiatry has always from a philosophical point of view been the *enfant terrible* of medicine, and today, more than ever, it is the battlefield of competing paradigms (Chapter 8). Some biologically minded psychiatrists accept the mechanical model of disease and regard mental disorders as physiological disturbances in the brain, others regard mental disorders as inappropriate behaviour which must be treated accordingly, and yet others stress that many psychiatric patients have existential problems which cannot be solved by the method of natural science. Those who adopt the last point of view may emphasize that it is necessary to understand the patient and to interpret his or her behaviour by means of psychoanalysis, and it will be shown in Chapter 11 that this approach is closely linked to the hermeneutic tradition of continental philosophy.

It will be remembered that, according to Kuhn, the paradigm of a science defines the legitimate area of research and also in this respect medical thinking has changed. Admittedly, doctors in the last century also concerned themselves with public health and the prevention of epidemics, but during recent years we have seen a wave of interest in epidemiology, industrial medicine and, especially, social medicine. The members of the medical profession who previously were mainly interested in the individual patient, are now directing their attention to those environmental and social factors which determine the development of disease, and in this border area between medicine and sociology important philosophical problems arise. The topic will be discussed in Chapter 10.

The new trends in medical thinking reflect a lack of confidence in modern medicine. The sceptical clinicians who established the critical clinical school doubted the efficacy of all the new drugs which were being introduced in the '60s, but since then more fundamental problems have attracted attention. Both the amount of research and the expenses of most health services have multiplied in the course of a few decades, but these efforts have not had the expected effect on morbidity and mortality in the developed world. We may have won the struggle against a large number of diseases, especially the infectious ones, but instead we are facing other health problems, especially degenerative diseases, malignant diseases and the so-called psychosomatic disorders, which are much more difficult to treat and at present impossible to prevent. Anybody who follows the development of medicine will know that progress continues in a large number of fields, but at the same time it is impossible to suppress the suspicion that the major health problems of the day cannot be solved within the conventional framework of ideas. The research activity is still intense, as medical research workers publish several hundred thousand scientific papers each year, but the medical journals also provide ample evidence that many research workers concern themselves with problems—or puzzles—of trifling importance, which have little or no connection with the health problems of modern society. Medical progress has not stopped but it seems to have lost its impetus, and an increasing number of doctors in many countries, who are worried about this state of affairs, are taking an interest in the philosophical basis of medical thinking. New journals on philosophy and ethics of medicine have appeared [9], and symposia are being held where doctors discuss philosophical topics.

Of course, the development of science cannot be viewed in isolation, and the recent developments in medicine reflect similar trends in society in general. That attitude which in medicine inspired the critical clinical school is no different from the one which in the political arena led to legislative measures against pollution and other ill-effects of new technologies. People have lost their naive belief in technological progress which—with intermissions—has characterized our culture since the industrial revolution, and instead they want to control the development. In other words, it is realized that new scientific results and new technologies are not an end in themselves, but only a means to improve life, and that realization must of necessity lead to a debate about moral values and, among doctors, to an interest in medical ethics.

The presentation in this chapter has been based on Kuhn's theories, and it cannot be denied that Kuhn assigns the individual scientist a somewhat passive role in the development of his science. The scientist is a puzzle-solver who accepts the ideas of his teachers, who is unable to analyse in detail the paradigm of his own science and who even disregards scientific results which do not tally with the established theories. To counteract this impression we shall finish this chapter by quoting some of the comments which the philosopher of science, Karl Popper, made in a discussion with Kuhn [10]. Popper accepts 'that we approach everything in the light of a preconceived theory' and that normal science, in Kuhn's sense, exists, but he believes that it is a danger to science and not a desirable state of affairs. He writes:

> In my view the 'normal' scientist, as Kuhn describes him, is a person one ought to be sorry for. ... I believe, and so do many others, that all teaching on the University level (and if possible below) should be training and encouragement in critical thinking. The 'normal' scientist, as described by Kuhn, has been badly taught. He has been taught in a dogmatic spirit: he is a victim of indoctrination.

Popper also maintains that science is an evolutionary rather than a revolutionary process and expresses this belief in the following way:

> I do admit that at any moment we are prisoners caught in the framework of our theories; our expectations, our past experience; our language. But, we are prisoners in a Pickwickean sense; if we try, we can break out of our framework at any time. Admittedly, we shall find ourselves again in a framework, but it will be a better and roomier one; and we can at any moment break out of it again.

In Popper's view the scientist does not only produce new knowledge within the established paradigm, as he is also co-responsible for the gradual adjustment of this paradigm. However, in the latter of the quotations Popper belittles the difficulties as he makes it sound as easy to change one's paradigm as to change one's overcoat. Popper is probably much too optimistic in this respect, but, if we did not agree just a little with his criticism of Kuhn, we should not have written this book. We do not regard the philosophy of medicine as a purely academic discipline, but believe that philosophical studies may help medical scientists and clinicians to solve the health problems of modern society.

Notes and references

1 Kuhn, T.S. *The Structure of Scientific Revolutions*, 2nd edn. Chicago: The University of Chicago Press, 1970.
2 The concept of tacit knowledge was introduced by Michael Polanyi in his book *Personal Knowledge. Towards a Post-Critical Philosophy*. London: Routledge and Kegan Paul, 1958.
3 In the first edition of his book, Kuhn does not attempt to define what is meant by a paradigm, and Margaret Masterman has pointed out that he used the word in at least twenty-two different ways (in: Lakatos, I. & Musgrave, A. (eds) *Criticism and the Growth of Knowledge*. London: Cambridge University Press, 1970, pp. 59–89). The cited paragraph is found in a postscript to the second edition of *The Structure of Scientific Revolutions* (p. 175) where Kuhn discusses the nature of the paradigm in greater detail.
4 p. 46 in [1].
5 p. 47 in [1].
6 p. 44 in [1].
7 Kuhn is quoting from Wittgenstein's *Philosophical Investigations*.
8 p. 80 in [1].
9 e.g. The *Journal of Medicine and Philosophy* and the *Journal of Medical Ethics*.
10 Popper, K. Normal science and its dangers. In: Lakatos, I. & Musgrave, A. (eds) *Criticism and the Growth of Knowledge*. London: Cambridge University Press, 1970, pp. 51–8.

CHAPTER 2
EMPIRICISM AND REALISM:
A PHILOSOPHICAL PROBLEM

*I*magine a room in a Cambridge college at the turn of the century, where a group of undergraduates are having their afternoon tea. The fire is dancing, the air is heavy with tobacco smoke, and the undergraduates, who are doing a course in philosophy, are debating the somewhat theoretical question, whether or not the cow in the meadow is still there when nobody is looking at it. In the following excerpt of their rather naive discussion the statements have been numbered for the sake of the subsequent comments.

1 'The cow is there,' said Ansell, lighting a match. 'She exists whether or not we are aware of her. She is there now.'

2 'You have not proved it,' said a voice. 'You cannot possibly know that you are right.'

3 Ansell frowned. 'What an unreasonable objection,' he retorted. 'Of course, I know she is there. I have proved it to myself. Whether I'm in Cambridge or Iceland or dead, the cow will be there.'

4 'You still have not proved it,' repeated the voice. 'I might just as well say that I have proved to myself that she is not there, that there is no cow at all.'

A discussion like this one takes place at the start of E. M. Forster's novel *The Longest Journey* [1], and it is relevant in the context of this book, as the points of view which are expressed by Ansell and the anonymous voice reflect the two great systems of thought, realism and empiricism [2], which for centuries have pervaded scientific thinking.

It is one of the purposes of this chapter to explain as simply as possible some of the most fundamental concepts of philosophy, and we ask the reader to bear with us, when on the next few pages we shall introduce a number of, presumably, unfamiliar philosophical terms. We shall have to use these terms (some of which are shown in Table 1) when in the following chapter we discuss the problems of medicine.

Table 1. Basic philosophical distinctions

Level of discussion	Philosophical positions	
Ontological	Realism	Anti-realism
Epistemological	Rationalism	Empiricism

The first important distinction is that between ontological and epistemological questions, and those who look up the meaning of these words in a dictionary will find explanations like these:

> **Ontology** (from Greek *on* = being) is the theory of being, and ontological questions are those which concern what there *is* in the world, what really *exists*, and what is the *true nature* of things.
> **Epistemology** (from Greek *episteme* = knowledge) is the theory of knowledge, and epistemological questions are those which concern what can be *known* about the world.

These explanations are correct, but difficult to grasp, and we shall try to illustrate the use of the words by means of the discussion about the cow in the meadow.

In the first statement Ansell declares that the cow *exists*, and that statement is obviously ontological. He is what philosophers call a realist, and he uses the cow to illustrate his belief in the independent existence of the material world. *Realism* is the ontological position that the external world is real, that it exists independently of us, and that it is the objects, structures and mechanisms of that world which stimulate our senses.

In the second statement, the 'voice' expresses his disagreement, but it is worth noticing that he does not say that Ansell is wrong and that the existence of the cow does depend on the fact that she is being observed. He only says that Ansell cannot *know* that he is right. In other words, the 'voice' does not make an ontological, but an epistemological claim. He is an empiricist, as he believes that only observed phenomena qualify as sources of knowledge, and he draws the radical conclusion from his belief that we cannot know anything about the existence of an unobserved cow. *Empiricism* is the epistemological position that ultimately all knowledge stems from sense experience.

In the third statement Ansell tries to counter this epistemological objection. Like all realists, he faces the problem that he cannot prove by means of his senses that he is right, and he resorts to the argument that it would be unreasonable to doubt the independent existence of the external world. He has arrived at this conclusion, not by the evidence of his senses, but by his reason or *ratio,* and therefore he is what philosophers call a rationalist. *Rationalism* can be defined as the epistemological position that, besides sense experience, reason is a source of knowledge. The justification of realism on the ontological level requires rationalism on the epistemological level.

In the fourth statement the 'voice' returns to the ontological problem. He still does not say that Ansell is wrong, but only that he might claim with the same degree of justification that there is no cow at all. What he means is that it is also possible, as some philosophers have asserted [3], that there is no external world and that an object like a cow is no more than a seemingly stable complex of sense impressions, which are not caused by anything outside our own minds. On the ontological level the 'voice' is an *anti-realist* in the sense that he professes complete agnosticism as regards ontological questions. Empiricism on the epistemological level is usually associated with anti-realism on the ontological level.

It is typical that those who discuss this classical philosophical dilemma are not on the same wavelength. The realist regards ontological questions as primary in relation to epistemological ones, and therefore he is not impressed by the empiricist who argues on the epistemological level. The empiricist, on the other hand, regards epistemological questions as the primary ones, as he holds that we must decide what can be known, before we consider what exists. Therefore, he is not convinced by the realist's ontological assumptions.

At this stage the reader may well be feeling that we are wasting his time by discussing the existence or non-existence of a cow, but, apart from the introduction of the terminology, there are two reasons why the discussion is important.

Firstly, empiricism has had an immense influence on modern science, and, as we shall discuss in the next chapter, it is possible to distinguish between realist and empiricist trends even in contemporary medicine. We shall describe how the realists among scientists try to find out what *really* goes on, for instance, in the human body, while the empiricists pay more attention to the statistical association between observed phenomena. We shall also show that the complete lack of interest in ontological and metaphysical [4] questions, which is one of the characteristics of empiricist thinking, is particularly pronounced in modern social medicine (Chapter 10).

Secondly, modern medicine presents important ontological questions. We do not really suggest that it is necessary for us to consider the *general* ontological question, whether or not there is an external world, but we shall have to consider in full earnest a number of *specific* ontological questions. To what extent is it reasonable to say that abstract entities like diseases exist (Chapter 6)? What is the true nature of mental disease (Chapter 8)? Is man just a biological organism, or is he more than that (Chapter 9)? Do moral values exist in the sense that they are part of the fabric of the world or are they no more than personal opinions (Chapter 12)? Are mental states essentially different from material objects and processes, or can they be reduced to neurophysiological states (Chapter 14)? Both the research methods which we choose and our attitude to clinical problems will to a considerable extent depend on our answers to such questions.

The empiricist position

The rise of empiricist philosophy in the 17th and 18th centuries can only be fully understood if it is seen in a historical perspective. The great thinkers of ancient Greece and medieval Europe had to a large extent concerned themselves with speculations about the nature of the world, the purpose of life and the existence of God, but following the scientific achievements of men like Kepler, Galileo, Harvey, Newton and Boyle, the intellectual climate changed, and both philosophers and scientists developed a sceptical attitude to ontological inquiries. They taught that one must rely entirely on the evidence of one's senses.

This school of thought is associated with a large number of well-known philosophers: John Locke (1632–1704), George Berkeley (1685–1753) and David Hume (1711–76) may be regarded as the founders of empiricism; Auguste Comte (1798–1857) championed similar ideas in France, and in this century the logical positivists of the Vienna Circle and their successors have analysed the logical consequences of empiricist thinking [5].

These philosophers have disagreed on a number of important points, but they have all shared the fundamental belief that all knowledge is derived from experience. In the following famous passage Locke asserts the empiricist creed by stating that the original state of mind is that of a *tabula rasa* (a blank slate) or a sheet of white paper:

> Let us suppose the mind to be, as we say, white paper, void of all characters, without any *ideas*; how comes it to be furnished? Whence comes it by that vast store, which the busy and boundless fancy of man has painted on it, with an almost endless variety? Whence has it all the materials of reason and knowledge? To this I answer, in one word, from *experience*: in that, all our knowledge is founded; and from that it ultimately derives itself [6].

Empiricists, of course, also accept the laws of logic and mathematics—and some have taken a particular interest in those disciplines—but they do not see this as an inconsistency in their theory. They assert that logical and mathematical deductions are analytic, which means that they do not generate new knowledge, but only serve to analyse existing knowledge.

John Locke did his very best to reconcile his empiricist beliefs with realism. He asserted that the mind at the beginning of life could be likened to 'a white paper', but he also claimed that our sensory impressions are caused by an external reality. According to Locke, our ideas must to some extent reflect the true nature of the things perceived, but this true nature—the real essence—remains unknown. Locke's philosophical theory is not fully consistent, as his belief in an external reality is founded on reason and not on experience, but, as we shall explain later, it may serve as a starting point for those who reject the extreme empiricist position. The analysis of the structure of the disease classification in Chapter 6 is to a large extent inspired by Locke's philosophy.

David Hume also struggled with this philosophical dilemma, and he was the first of the empiricist philosophers to draw the ultimate logical consequence of his empiricist belief. He claimed, as the true empiricist must do, that we simply cannot know what causes our perceptions—if they are caused—but he also had the intellectual honesty to confess that in our daily lives we have to accept that the cows in the meadow and the trees in our garden are real. In the *Treatise of Human Nature* he writes:

> Thus the sceptic still continues to reason and believe, even tho' he asserts, that he cannot defend his reason by reason... We may well ask, *what causes induce us to believe in the existence of body?* but 'tis in vain to ask, *whether there be body or not?* That is a point, which we must take for granted in all our reasonings [7].

The ontological scepticism of empiricists like Hume (and the 'voice') is hard to accept when we are talking about cows in the meadow, but it is a bit more acceptable in advanced science. Scientists do not concern themselves with the observation of cows and trees, but use ingenious instruments to study natural phenomena which are not directly observable. As the result of complicated experiments, medical scientists have postulated the existence of specific receptors on the surface of brain cells, just as physicists have postulated the existence of photons and positrons, and it is not quite unreasonable to ask whether such entities really exist or whether they are creations of the scientists' imagination, which only serve to organize their ideas.

Even medical practitioners do not rely on direct observation. They use *sense-extending* instruments [8], like X-ray equipment and microscopes, which permit them to perceive things which they would otherwise be unable to perceive; they employ *detecting instruments*, like the electrocardiograph, which permit them to detect otherwise imperceptible phenomena; and they do complicated chemical analyses which reveal the composition of the examined objects. By indirect means they create a picture of reality which they cannot directly perceive.

The anti-realism of the empiricists has the unfortunate effect that it proves necessary to redefine concepts like *causality, laws of nature* and *objectivity* in such a way that they do not presuppose a reality beyond our observations.

In ordinary language, the statement that A causes B means that A helps to generate B through some mechanism or other, but this *generative theory of causality* is, of course, quite unacceptable to empiricists as it implies that the causal reaction takes place in the external world independently of our observations. Instead they claim that the statement that A causes B only means that phenomenon B succeeds phenomenon A in a regular manner. According to this alternative theory, which is called the *succession theory* or the *Humean theory of causality*, the idea of causation is explained in psychological terms. If we observe time and time again that B follows A, then we learn to expect B when A has occurred, and the causal relationship is no more than this expectation. It is, to quote Hume, a *mental habit*, which we erroneously extrapolate to an external world. The succession theory may be refined by analysing in great detail the logical relationship between causes and effects, and we shall show the usefulness of such analyses, when we discuss the causation of disease in Chapter 5.

Laws of nature are treated in much the same way. The famous physicist, Ernst Mach (1838–1916), who was an extreme empiricist, stated that laws of nature do not tell us what really goes on in the world, but that their function is the 'mnemonic reproduction of facts in mind' [9]; they are no more than mental constructions that serve to describe as concisely as possible the observations which we have made. Mach claimed, for instance, that Galileo's laws of falling bodies were 'simple and compendious directions for reproducing in thought all possible motions of falling bodies'.

Objectivity is yet another important term which is used by empiricists in a very restricted sense. Usually, this word has ontological implications, as a phenomenon is said to be objective, if it is believed to exist independently of the observer, but empiricists, who of course cannot accept this interpretation, equate objectivity with *inter-subjectivity*. If an observer, looking out of the window, sees a cow, and if other observers with a normal faculty of vision make exactly the same observation, then the observation statement that there is a cow in the meadow, is said to be objective, meaning that it is inter-subjective, public or *verifiable* by others.

We have characterized empiricism as a rebellion against speculative thinking, and the logical positivists of this century, in particular Carnap (1891–1970), have tried to formulate a

demarcation criterion which may serve to distinguish those propositions which are meaningful from those which are not. They chose the *criterion of verifiability,* according to which only those statements which in principle are verifiable can be labelled as meaningful. To explain this idea, let us consider the following statements:
1 There is a cow in the meadow.
2 The patient's right knee is swollen.
3 There are large oil deposits in Greenland under the inland ice.
4 The patient has a myocardial infarction.
5 These oysters taste well.
6 It is morally wrong not to tell the patient the truth about the diagnosis.

The first two statements are meaningful, as they can be verified—or falsified—by observation. So are the third and the fourth statements, as they are also, in principle, verifiable, even though it may not actually be feasible to explore that part of the Greenlandic underground or to inspect directly the patient's heart muscle. The last two propositions, on the other hand, are not regarded as meaningful, as it is impossible to imagine an observation which may serve to determine whether they are true or false; they only reflect the subjective feelings of the individuals who made them. Probably, most people will agree that it is not worthwhile spending a lot of time discussing the taste of oysters, but it is one of the more serious consequences of the verifiability criterion that all attempts to discuss moral issues rationally are considered equally futile. This nihilistic attitude to moral philosophy, which is called emotivism, will be discussed in Chapter 13.

The verifiability criterion, however, also leads to other difficulties. Firstly, it has been pointed out with some justification that the criterion defeats itself. It is not itself verifiable, and therefore it must by empiricist standards be regarded as meaningless. Secondly, the criterion may well be applicable to *singular* statements (e.g. this patient has a swollen knee), but scientists usually concern themselves with *general* statements (e.g. all patients with a gastric ulcer produce gastric acid), and such statements cannot be verified with absolute certainty by experience alone. This is the classical *problem of induction,* which we shall briefly explain.

From the empiricist's point of view the scientific process starts

Empiricism and Realism: A Philosophical Problem 21

with observation. The gastroenterologist observes again and again that patients with a gastric ulcer produce hydrochloric acid in their stomachs, and in the end they conclude that this is a universal law ('no acid, no ulcer'), but this leap from experience, which always consists of singular observations, to a 'law of nature' cannot be defended logically, as it can never be excluded that the next patient will prove the law to be false. Ornithologists for a long time believed that 'all swans are white', but the first explorers to reach the Australian continent made them change their minds.

This logical problem has vexed empiricist philosophers ever since the days of David Hume, and there can be no doubt that it challenges the very basis of their thinking. Empiricist philosophers, who believe that it is impossible for scientists to discover what the world is really like, have asserted that it is the sole aim of all scientific efforts to establish 'laws of nature' which may predict what will happen in the future, but because of the problem of induction such predictions can never be regarded as certain.

The riddle of induction may also be formulated in a different way. Predictions of future occurrences which are founded on past experience presuppose the principle that the future will reflect the past, and it is impossible for the empiricist to justify his belief in this principle. True enough, we have often observed in the past that our predictions held true, but we cannot predict from that experience that the same will be the case in the future, as that prediction presupposes the very principle which we wish to justify. It is not much of a logical argument to claim that past experience shows that past experience is reliable.

Empiricists may, of course, try to defend themselves by claiming that laws of nature which have been confirmed again and again may not be absolutely true, but that they are very nearly true, and that predictions from such laws possess at least a high degree of probability. It will, however, be explained in Chapter 7 that it is difficult to state in objective terms what is meant by the probability of the truth of a hypothesis, and, apart from that, probabilistic predictions about future occurrences also presuppose that the future will reflect the past.

The riddle of induction has been attacked with renewed enthusiasm by the logical positivists of this century, but as yet it has proved impossible to defend in logical terms the jump from singular observation statements to general theory. Bertrand Russell simply concludes that 'induction is an independent logical principle, incapable of being inferred either from experience or from other logical principles, and that without this principle science is impossible' [10].

Popper's solution

Karl Popper (b. 1902) is probably the most influential philosopher of science of this century, and many scientists, even those who do not usually read books on philosophy, are acquainted with the basic principles of his views of science. The popularity of Popper's philosophy is due partly to the fact that it has been well explained in simple terms by, among others, Bryan Magee [11] and the medical Nobel prize winner Peter Medawar [12].

Popper makes the very important point that the empiricists put the cart in front of the horse when they claim that science proceeds from observation to theory, since there is no such thing as a pure observation which does not depend on theory. Popper writes:

> ... the belief that we can start with pure observations alone, without anything in the nature of a theory, is absurd; as may be illustrated by the story of the man who dedicated his life to natural science, wrote down everything he could observe, and bequeathed his priceless collection of observations to the Royal Society to be used as inductive evidence....
>
> Observation is always selective. It needs a chosen object, a definite task, an interest, a point of view, a problem [13].

The first step in the scientific process is not observation, but the generation of a hypothesis which may then be tested critically by observations and experiments.

Popper also makes the important claim that the goal of the scientist's efforts is not the verification but the *falsification* of the initial hypothesis. As explained above, it is logically impossible to verify the truth of a general law by repeated observation, but, at least in principle, it is possible to falsify such a law by a single observation. Repeated observations of white swans did not prove that all swans are white, but the observation of a single black swan sufficed to falsify that general statement [14].

On the basis of these ideas Popper expounds his views on science.

Empiricism and Realism: A Philosophical Problem

The scientist must be creative, he must be able to develop original ideas and to make novel and bold conjectures, which he then does his very best to falsify by critical experimentation. To Popper this procedure is much more than the correct scientific method; it is a way of life:

> Assume that we have deliberately made it our task to live in this unknown world of ours; to adjust ourselves to it as well as we can; to take advantage of the opportunities we can find in it; and to explain it, if possible . . . *then there is no more rational procedure than the method of trial and error—of conjecture and refutation*; of boldly proposing theories; of trying our best to show that these are erroneous; and of accepting them tentatively if our critical efforts are unsuccessful [15].

The empiricists used the criterion of verifiability to distinguish between those statements which are meaningful and those which are not, and in much the same way Popper uses the *criterion of falsifiability* to distinguish between those theories which fall within the province of science and those which may be labelled pseudoscientific. As examples of the latter category Popper mentions astrology and his two pet aversions: psychoanalysis and Marxism. Those who read the horoscopes in the evening press will agree that the predictions are usually worded so carefully that they are bound to come true, whatever happens. They are almost tautological, like the statement that it will either rain or not rain tomorrow, and therefore they are not falsifiable; they are pseudoscientific. We shall not in this book discuss Popper's views of Marxist political philosophy, but we shall consider his views of psychoanalysis in Chapter 11.

Popper's philosophy of science has great immediate appeal to the critical scientist, but it also has its shortcomings. The criterion of falsifiability is simple, and its importance from a logical point of view is indisputable, but in practice it is not easy to handle. Firstly, Popper himself points out that there is no such thing as a pure, neutral observation and, therefore, the scientist who makes an experiment which contradicts a theory cannot be sure whether the theory has been falsified or whether the observation (or the experimental set-up) was at fault. In practice, he will have to repeat the observation and alter the experimental conditions before he gives up his theory. Secondly, medical scientists do not often concern themselves with absolute statements like 'all swans are white' but with relative ones like 'duodenal ulcer patients on average produce more acid than normal subjects', and the results of investigations of such problems are rarely unambiguous. The scientist will have to subject his observations to a statistical analysis, and, as we shall discuss in Chapter 7, the final decision will depend not only on the observations, but also on convention as regards the choice of statistical tests and the accepted level of significance [16].

Popper claims that he has solved the problem of induction, but it would be more correct to say that he has tried to bypass the problem, and it is doubtful to what extent it is permissible to do so. There can be no doubt that scientists in many cases attempt to falsify hypotheses, but in other cases they do reason inductively. One of the authors of this book once used histochemical techniques to study the metabolism of white blood cells and, among other things, he wanted to find out whether or not granulocytes contain a particular enzyme, glycogen synthetase. He simply wanted to answer this question and did not hypothesize in advance that granulocytes possess the enzyme or that they do not possess it. He succeeded in demonstrating the enzyme in a sample of his own leucocytes and, to be sure, he repeated the experiment a few times. Then, he did the same experiment on a few other persons, confirmed the result and published a paper with the conclusion: human granulocytes contain glycogen synthetase. This simple study fits Popperian thinking in so far as the observations were not theory-free, but it is very difficult to see that he tried to falsify a particular hypothesis. Instead, he concluded by induction from a very small number of experiments that human granulocytes in general contain that enzyme.

Medical papers also contain numerous statistical calculations which reflect inductive reasoning. A clinician may correlate the serum creatinine and the serum urea in a number of patients, and the regression line which illustrates graphically the association between the two variables may be regarded as a law of nature (in the empiricist sense) which has been inferred from a series of observations. Even such a simple measure as the mean survival time of patients with a particular disease is based on inductive reasoning, and the clinician who tries to estimate the 'true' five-year survival rate, by calculating the confidence interval (Chapter 7), makes an inductive inference.

The falsification principle is not problem-free, and the problem of induction has not been solved.

The realist alternative

Empiricist philosophers taught scientists the importance of empirical evidence, but from a purely philosophical point of view radical empiricism seems to lead to a dead end. It creates logical problems which cannot be solved, and it imposes upon us a view of the world which is at least counter-intuitive.

In order to trace where things went wrong, we must go all the way back to Locke. He was a realist in so far as he believed in the existence of the external world, but he was also an empiricist as he believed that *all* knowledge is derived from experience, and notwithstanding its immediate attraction, this point of view is not fully consistent. Later empiricists who tried to solve this dilemma by denouncing realism were unsuccessful, so instead we shall have to weaken the empiricist position.

One eminent philosopher, who has reasoned somewhat along these lines, was Immanuel Kant (1724–1804). Kant admired Hume, who, he said, woke him from his dogmatic slumbers, but he did not accept the empiricist idea, first expressed by Locke, that the mind was originally like a blank sheet of paper. To use a very modern analogy, Kant's picture of the original state of the mind was more like that of a computer which has not yet received any input, but which has been programmed to organize all the information which it will later receive. According to Kant, space and time are preconditions for the perception of something as an object, and human beings have been 'programmed' to think in categories of quantity, quality, causality, possibility, necessity, existence, etc. Our picture of the world reflects both this *a priori* organization of our perceptions and our actual observations. Kant is a *rationalist* as he asserts that our empirical knowledge is organized according to *a priori* principles, but, like the empiricists, he is a sceptic as regards our ability to know what the world is really like. We cannot know the things-in-themselves.

Contemporary philosophers and psychologists have also given

up the idea that the mind was originally a 'blank sheet of paper' and deny that there is such a thing as a pure observation. We have already presented Popper's and Kuhn's views of the matter, and here we shall illustrate the theory-dependence of observations with a medical example.

Imagine that a layman and a skilled pathologist were asked to look through the microscope at the same histological preparation. The layman would probably describe the shape of the preparation ('it looks a bit like a flag which is torn at one end') and its colour ('it is like red marble, and there are some blue dots at that corner!'), but he would not be able to make head or tail of the observations. The pathologist, on the other hand, would immediately recognize the architecture of liver tissue, and he would also notice at once that there was something seriously wrong: the normal sharp demarcation between the portal spaces and the liver lobules has disappeared, granulocytes are emigrating from the portal spaces in between the liver cells, and in some areas the liver cells are seen to be dying or dead. In this formalin-fixed thin slice of tissue he would see a liver which was gradually being destroyed and he would diagnose a chronic active hepatitis. Of course, the layman and the pathologist were exposed to the same visual stimulus, but when such a stimulus becomes conscious it is already imbibed with theory. The two observers did not see the same thing, did not make the same observation.

Empiricist philosophy must, of course, be viewed in a historical perspective. The metaphysical theories before the era of enlightenment had been much too extravagant, and it was only natural that the empiricists felt that science must start afresh with systematic observations and the establishment of descriptive laws of nature. In Chapter 6 we shall quote Locke for having stated that 'our knowledge of the real essence of the things observed is as small as a countryman's knowledge of the works of the clock at Strassbourg', and at that time the statement was both justified and true. Today, however, it would be absurd to maintain that we have no knowledge of the real world. We may agree with Popper that we can never be quite sure that our theories are true, but the efficacy of modern technology, which at least to some extent is based on scientific theories, proves beyond doubt that we have in some areas reached what Popper calls 'an approximation to the truth'.

Empiricism and Realism: A Philosophical Problem 27

The development of modern science is inextricably bound up with empiricist philosophy, but both philosophical reflection and the results of science suggest the conclusion that the empiricist position is not tenable. On the *ontological level* we shall therefore accept the realist's point of view that it is the purpose of science to explore what really goes on in the world, and on the *epistemological* level we shall deny that observations constitute the only source of knowledge; pure observations do not exist. Therefore, we shall also reject the view that causation is no more than the succession of observed events and that laws of nature only describe the regularity of observations. A causal relationship exists, if one event generates another event through some mechanism or other, and it is these mechanisms which follow the laws of nature. Causal relationships and laws of nature are objective in the sense that they exist independently of our observations.

The realist position does not solve the logical problem of induction, but knowledge of the underlying mechanisms sometimes makes the problem less troublesome. The gambler who has won five times running at the roulctte wheel will be ill-advised to infer from this experience that he will go on winning, but the scientist who infers from his observations on five people that everybody's granulocytes contain glycogen is not equally foolish. It is well established that all (healthy) human beings have granulocytes in their blood, that the cells play an important part in the defence mechanism of the body, that these functions require energy and that this energy is released by the breakdown of glycogen. Glycogen synthetase mediates the formation of glycogen, and therefore it is not likely that the presence of that enzyme in the granulocytes of five people is a chance finding. It fits so well with existing theory that it is reasonable to assume that the enzyme is part of the general picture. The general statement that human granulocytes contain glycogen synthetase is not only the result of inductive inference; it is also based on existing theoretical knowledge.

The philosophy of science has for a long time been dominated by empiricist thinking, but during the last few decades philosophers like J. J. C. Smart, R. Harré, I. Hacking and R. Bhaskar have argued in favour of a realist theory of science [17-20]. Bhaskar writes that it is necessary to come to terms with the fundamental paradox of all science:

... that men in their social activity produce knowledge which is a social product much like any other, which is no more independent of its production and the men who produce it than motor cars, armchairs and books ... and which is no less subject to change than any other commodity. This is one side of 'knowledge'. The other is that knowledge is '*of*' things which are not produced by men at all: the specific gravity of mercury, the process of electrolysis, the mechanism of light propagation. None of these 'objects of knowledge' depend upon human activity. If men ceased to exist sound would continue to travel and heavy bodies fall to earth in exactly the same way, though *ex hypothesi* there would be no one to know it [20].

In this way scientific knowledge has both a transitive and an intransitive aspect. Knowledge in the form of a scientific theory must be regarded as a changeable social product, and as such it is *transitive*, but the object of that knowledge, which does not depend on our existence, is *intransitive*.

This distinction is important as it reveals the deficiencies of different views of science. Naive realists, for instance, who believe that the world is just as we imagine it to be, disregard the transitive aspect of scientific knowledge, whereas empiricists, who deny that we can obtain certain knowledge of the external world, disregard the intransitive aspect. A balanced theory of natural science must take into account both aspects and the relationship between them.

Notes and references

1 This is not a literal citation from Forster's book, as we have permitted ourselves to sharpen the arguments a little.
2 This dichotomy is debatable, as empiricism is not the only philosophical theory which is opposed to realism. However, we only wish to introduce the reader to two important traditions in scientific thinking.
3 The theories of Bishop George Berkeley (1685–1753) and the Austrian physicist Ernst Mach (1838–1916) come close to that ontological position, which is called phenomenalism.
4 Metaphysics (from *meta* = after, beyond, and *phusis* = nature) is the investigation of all that which lies beyond the reach of ordinary experience. It has wider connotations than ontology, but often the two words are used synonymously. It is a result of the influence of empiricist thinking that the word *metaphysical* in modern speech is usually used disparagingly in the sense 'obscure' or 'supernatural'.

Empiricism and Realism: A Philosophical Problem 29

5 e.g. Moritz Schlick, Otto Neurath and Rudolf Carnap, who were members of the influential Vienna Circle which met regularly in the 1920s and '30s. Among their successors or sympathizers may be mentioned Bertrand Russell, A. J. Ayer, C. G. Hempel, W. V. O. Quine and B. van Fraasen.

6 Locke, J. *An Essay Concerning Human Understanding* (originally published 1690), ed. P. H. Nidditch. Oxford: Oxford University Press, 1975, Book II, Chapter I, § 2, p. 104.

7 Hume, D. *A Treatise of Human Nature* (originally published 1739), ed. L. A. Selby-Brigge. Oxford: Clarendon Press, 1964, Book I, Part IV, Section II, p. 187.

8 Harré, R. *The Philosophies of Science*. Oxford University Press, 1972, p. 19.

9 Mach, E. *The Science of Mechanics*. Cited by Harré [8].

10 Russell, B. *History of Western Philosophy*. 2nd edn. London: George Allen & Unwin, 1961, p. 647.

11 Magee, B. *Popper*. Fontana Collins, 1973.

12 Medawar, P.B. *Induction and Intuition in Scientific Thought*. Philadelphia: American Philosophical Society, 1969.

13 Popper, K.R. *Conjectures and Refutations*. 2nd edn. London: Routledge and Kegan Paul, 1965, p. 46.

14 Scientists do not like to have their favourite hypothesis falsified, and, as Popper points out, they tend to 'immunize' their hypotheses by modifying either their definitions or the hypotheses themselves when they see the test results. An ornithologist, who wanted to maintain that all swans are white, might claim that black swans are not swans at all, or that the hypothesis that swans outside the Australian continent are white has not been falsified. 'If we allow such immunization, then every theory becomes unfalsifiable' (Popper, K. *Unended Quest. An Intellectual Autobiography*. Fontana Collins, 1976, p. 42).

15 p. 51 in [13].

16 Popper himself emphasizes that the falsification of a theory is not simply the result of a confrontation between the theory and an observation. He writes: 'From a logical point of view, the testing of a theory depends upon basic statements whose acceptance or rejection, in its turn, depends upon our *decisions*. Thus it is *decisions* which settle the fate of theories' (Popper, K.R. *The Logic of Scientific Discovery*. 2nd edn. London: Hutchinson, 1968, p. 108).

17 Smart, J.J.C. *Philosophy and Scientific Realism*. London: Routledge and Kegan Paul, 1963.

18 Harré, R. *The Principles of Scientific Thinking*. London: Macmillan, 1970.

19 Hacking, I. *Representing and Intervening*. London: Cambridge University Press, 1983.

20 Bhaskar, R. *A Realist Theory of Science*. London: Harvester Press, 1975, p. 21.

CHAPTER 3
EMPIRICISM AND REALISM: TWO OPPOSING TRENDS IN MEDICAL THINKING

*E*mpiricism and realism are philosophical positions, and we do not wish to suggest that there are two varieties of medicine, a purely empiricist one and a purely realist one. It is, however, possible to discern both empiricist and realist trends in medical thinking, and in this chapter we wish to show the importance of this distinction. We shall discuss briefly the historical background and we shall consider conflicting tendencies in contemporary medical thought.

Speculative realism

Superficially, there are many similarities between medical practice in the 17th and 18th centuries and today. Also in those days most doctors were respected members of society, and they did their best to help those patients who sought their advice. They did not examine the patients as we do today, but they listened to their complaints and prescribed those remedies which they believed would be most effective. If, however, we could ask them how they made their diagnoses and why they believed that their remedies were effective, their answers would have made us feel the distance in time. Medical theory, two or three centuries ago, was still to a large extent based on mere speculation, and we should find it very hard to understand their explanations—and even harder to accept them.

Many clinicians still accepted Hippocratic humoral pathology with its distinction between four 'humours' with different qualities:

blood (which is hot and moist), phlegm (which is cold and moist), yellow bile (which originates in the liver and is hot and dry), and black bile (which is formed in the spleen and is cold and dry). They believed that these humours were properly balanced in healthy persons and that disease followed, if the balance was upset. By inspecting the patient they could 'diagnose' the nature of the disturbance, and they had different remedies for sanguinary, phlegmatic, bilious and melancholic states. Patients with acute infections were often diagnosed as being sanguinary, and in such cases blood letting was the logical treatment.

Eighteenth century medicine was characterized by a lively competition between different schools of thought, and other theories were equally popular. William Cullen (1712–90), who held the chair of medicine in Edinburgh and was known as an inspiring teacher, taught that all vital processes are regulated by the central nervous system and that illness is mainly a nervous disorder. In febrile conditions the energy of the brain is weakened, and the resulting atony manifests itself as general fatigue, chills, pallor and a weak pulse. As a reaction, the peripheral arteries contract in a spasm, which is transmitted to the heart and produces a quick pulse. The therapist must moderate the reaction by removing the irritants, including the contents of the stomach and gut, and emetics and laxatives were regarded as logical remedies. The spasm must be relieved by blood letting, and the atony itself could be counteracted with tonics [1].

The humoral pathologists and Cullen were realists as they believed in the existence of an underlying disease mechanism, and they were rationalists to an extravagant degree as they also believed that it was possible by armchair reasoning alone to ascertain the nature of that disease mechanism. To the modern doctor these theories simply make no sense, but it is worth remembering that even today millions of patients all over the world are treated according to the speculative theories of local traditional medicine and unorthodox therapeutic schools.

Homeopathy is a good example of a well-established unorthodox therapeutic school which is as speculative as humoral pathology. Samuel Hahnemann, its founder, accepted as self-evident that every powerful drug induces a specific kind of disease and that naturally occurring diseases can be cured by giving the patient a small dose of that drug which produces that particular disease. This doctrine, called *similia similibus curantur*, is still taught at a number of colleges of homeopathy, and it does not seem to worry homeopaths at all that they sometimes use drugs in such weak concentrations that each dose on average contains less than one molecule of the 'active' substance.

However, it must also be remembered that ontological theories, which are now rejected as figments of the imagination, sometimes brought about genuine advances in medicine. Alchemy led to the introduction of mercury treatment for syphilis, and William Harvey, who discovered the circulation of the blood, was guided by the mediaeval idea that man is a microcosm in the macrocosm of the universe. In his book *De motu cordis* of 1628, Harvey characterizes the heart as the sun of the universe, and he writes explicitly that the idea of the circular motion of blood was inspired by the circular motion of celestial bodies [2].

Nevertheless, it is no good denying that most of the therapeutic remedies which doctors used two hundred years ago had no beneficial effects whatsoever, and that some of the most popular treatments were sometimes harmful. Digitalis treatment of 'the dropsy', fresh fruit for the prevention of scurvy and vaccination against smallpox have proved their worth, but these are rare exceptions, and blood letting of dehydrated cholera patients, which was recommended well into the 19th century, is a good example of a practice which must have had disastrous effects. Of course, doctors at that time also attached great importance to experience, but, probably, they were satisfied to see that most of their patients survived; they did not ask themselves whether the patients would have survived anyway or whether some survived in spite of the treatment, and they certainly did not try to verify or falsify their speculative theories empirically.

Realism under empirical control

The scientific revolution in medicine did not occur until the beginning of the 19th century, when speculative realism finally gave way to a new kind of realism *which was subject to empirical control*. At that time, French pathologists developed an anatomical theory of disease, as they identified disease entities with anatomical lesions, and, unlike their predecessors, they did not content themselves with armchair reasoning. They performed meticulous studies at the autopsy table and related their anatomical findings to those clinical observations which they made before the patients died. Later that century, another generation of medical scientists developed a physiological theory as they regarded disease processes as functional disturbances, and they, too, tested their ideas by research in the laboratory. This development will be discussed in greater detail in Chapter 6, but in this context it is important to note that laboratory-oriented medical scientists, whether they adopted an anatomical, a physiological, a biochemical, a microbiological or some other point of view, were philosophical realists as they aimed at discovering the mechanisms of disease. They tested their theories and hypotheses empirically, but as pointed out in Chapter 2, theory always preceded observation. The end-result of these efforts was the biological concept of disease (see Chapter 4), which combines all these theories, but excludes all theory formation which cannot be tested empirically. Disease entities are now defined by a mixture of anatomical, physiological, microbiological and other criteria, and this conceptual heterogeneity is the strength rather than the weakness of contemporary medical thinking. The mechanical model constitutes a *transitive* human construction (see p. 28), but the fact that many of its components can be tested within different conceptual frameworks, under a variety of experimental conditions, helps to ensure that it reflects at least some aspects of *intransitive* reality.

Early empiricist trends

The empiricist demand for careful observation had some effects on medical thinking as early as the 17th century. Thomas Sydenham, who was a brilliant clinical observer and a personal friend of John Locke, stressed the importance of clinical observations at the bedside and described a number of disease entities on the basis of their clinical manifestations; his description of a disease like gout could be used in any modern textbook of medicine. He is also said to have distrusted the theories of his time, but in spite of that he remained a firm believer in the doctrines of Hippocratic humoral pathology.

In the 18th century, botanists worked out elaborate botanical taxonomies, and some, who were also physicians, attempted to classify diseases like plants. François Boissier de Sauvages wrote *Nosologia methodica,* which subdivides 'diseases' into ten classes, 295 genera and 2400 species; and the most famous of botanical taxonomists, the Swede Linnaeus, composed a *Genera morborum.* These disease classifications were undoubtedly inspired by empiricist thinking as no attention was paid to the disease mechanism. They were, in fact, no more than divisions and subdivisions of ill-defined symptoms, and they had no lasting effect on the development of modern medicine.

The anatomists, physiologists and bacteriologists of the last century were also influenced by empiricist philosophy in so far as they paid great attention to their empirical observations in the laboratory, but they were not empiricists. Medical scientists are realists, as they try to discover the mechanisms of disease, whereas the true empiricist denies that this is possible.

In the 1830s and '40s, however, time was ripe for a new mode of thought, which had much more in common with philosophical empiricism, and the schism between a realist and an empiricist trend in medical thinking, which has persisted to this day, took its beginning.

In those days, morbid anatomy, at least on the macroscopical level, was almost as developed as today, and laboratory-orientated scientists were beginning to take an interest in physiology, but as yet the influence of this type of research on clinical practice was almost nil. Medical treatment was still to a large extent based on the old Hippocratic theories, and the feeling of despondency which prevailed among clinicians in the 1830s is well expressed by the following quotation from the newly started *Danish Medical Journal* [3]:

> The Newton of medicine has not yet appeared, and unfortunately we may fear ... that we shall never see the genius who will convey that to medicine which physics found in algebra and which chemistry found in a pair of scales. Medicine is still what those sciences were a hundred years ago, a collection of unconnected theses.

Critical clinicians were at long last beginning to suspect that most of the things which they did for their patients were of no avail,

Empiricism and Realism in Medical Thinking

and they felt the need for meticulous observations, not only in the laboratory, but also at the bedside. A decade earlier, the first well-known continental empiricist philosopher, Auguste Comte, had delivered a series of lectures in Paris, in which he gave a historical account of human intellectual development and claimed that man must learn to rely only on positive facts, and it is possible that it was Comte's *positivism* which inspired a number of critical French doctors, especially Jules Gavaret and P. C. A. Louis.

Gavaret, too, gave a series of lectures, in which he analysed medical problems from an empiricist point of view, and in 1840 he published his remarkable book *Principes Généraux de Statistique Médicale* [4]. It is the forerunner of a completely new approach to clinical medicine, which was going to have far-reaching consequences more than a century later, and Gavaret deserves that we quote those ten tenets *in extenso*, in which he summarizes his views:

1 The Laws of Logic are insufficient for judging the effect of a given treatment for a given disease, and they are insufficient for ranking those treatments which are recommended for the same disease according to the degree of their effect.

2 These two important problems can only be solved by means of the Law of Large Numbers, which is applicable to therapeutic investigations.

3 The death rate which is obtained by statistical calculations is never a precise and correct expression of the effect of the treatment in question, but, the larger the number of observations, the closer the approximation.

4 A Therapeutic Law, obtained by comparing small numbers of facts, may be so far from the truth that it can never be trusted.

5 A Therapeutic Law is never absolute, but must always be expressed as a range. The range decreases when the number of observations increases, and its width can be determined by those numbers on which the statistical calculations are based.

6 In order to prefer one therapeutic method to another, the results must not only be better, but the difference must exceed a certain limit which depends on the number of cases.

7 If a difference does not reach this limit, which is low when the number of investigations is large, it can be ignored and regarded as non-existent.

8 The same rules and the same conclusions are applicable to the solution of problems in connection with the theory of epidemic constitutions.

9 One must follow the same rules in order to ascertain whether the death rate in a disease varies according to age, sex and location.

10 In investigations of aetiological problems, the Law of Large Numbers only serves to prove the presence or absence of an assumed specific cause, regardless of its nature. One must seek to determine the cause itself by means of considerations of a different order. This last question is outside the domain of statistics.

Already in the first three tenets Gavaret introduces the empiricist theme. Doctors must not base their therapeutic decisions on speculative theories and logical deduction, but they must study as many patients as possible and count the numbers of those who die and those who survive. In other words, they must discard theory and rely on positive facts. In tenets 4 and 5 Gavaret uses the expression 'a therapeutic law', and by that he simply means the death rate or cure rate in a sample of patients who have received a particular treatment; to the empiricist the demonstration of a law of nature is no more than the demonstration of a regular association between observed phenomena. In tenet 5 Gavaret also reminds us that the precision of such a statistical law of nature depends on the number of patients and that it is necessary to calculate what statisticians nowadays call confidence limits. According to tenets 6 and 7 we must distinguish between association by chance and true association, and we must disregard differences between treatment effects which are not, in our terminology, statistically significant. In the 8th and 9th tenets Gavaret states that the same principles must be applied when we wish to study the association between the incidence of a disease and environmental factors (the theory of epidemic constitutions), or the correlation between the death rate of a disease and demographic data. However, in the 10th tenet Gavaret suddenly beats a retreat from radical empiricism. Statistics only serve to establish the presence or absence of a causal factor, *regardless of its nature*. So, in spite of everything, a causal relationship is more than a regular succession of events and there is room for 'considerations of a different order'.

The modern reader may feel that Gavaret's tenets are somewhat trivial as they are little different from the recommendations of present-day statisticians, but that is exactly the point. Gavaret was more than a century ahead of his time, and his influence among his contemporaries was limited. A few doctors, both in France and abroad, tried to live up to his ideas, and the most famous of these, Pierre-Charles-Alexandre Louis (1787–1872), engaged himself in a crusade against those of his colleagues who treated their patients with the application of leeches and repeated venesections. In his *Recherches sur les Effets de la Saignée* [5] he managed to show, by means of statistical considerations, that blood-letting did not have the assumed beneficial effects, and gradually this age-old therapeutic practice was abandoned.

However, most of Gavaret's contemporaries ignored his advice, and perhaps that was only to be expected. He had suggested a method for comparing the effect of different treatments, but he lived at a time when there were few effective treatments to compare. Instead, the vast majority of those doctors who were interested in science continued to explore the mechanisms of disease, in the hope that one day they would possess so much knowledge that it would be possible to deduce the correct treatment in the individual patient by means of the 'Laws of Logic'.

Gavaret's ideas were premature but they were not completely forgotten, and after the Second World War the time was ripe for their revival in the form of the new *critical clinical school* (p. 8). At that time, the combination of new scientific knowledge, new technology and strong commercial interests resulted in an explosive development of new therapeutic and diagnostic remedies, which had to be tested critically in accordance with Gavaret's tenets.

Medical thinking today

Those days have passed when it was reasonable to query the justification of realism in medicine. It was always somewhat absurd to doubt the real existence of the cow in the meadow (Chapter 2), and today it is equally unreasonable to doubt that the heart is a pump which makes the blood circulate to all parts of the body, that the pancreas produces insulin which, through complex mechanisms, lowers the blood glucose, and that bacteria and viruses may invade the body, which then defends itself by means of phagocytes and the production of antibodies.

The realist approach pervades contemporary medical thinking. As an example, the teacher who gives a lecture on bronchial asthma will describe the symptoms and signs of asthmatic patients, but he will also give an account of the underlying mechanism. He may explain that in allergic asthma specific allergens produce mast cell degranulation, and that the substances which are released produce bronchial spasms, and he may conclude that the logical treatment of patients suffering from this condition comprises the elimination of allergens from the environment, treatment with powerful bronchodilators, and the inhalation of cromoglycate which inhibits the release of the active substances. Superficially, there is no great difference between the presentation of Cullen's fever theory on page 31 and this presentation of the modern asthma theory as, in both cases, we describe the disease mechanism and deduce the logical treatment, but of course the resemblance is only apparent. Cullen's theory was to a large extent the result of armchair reasoning, whereas the asthma theory is the only one which fits a multitude of carefully executed experiments. Those who wish to probe the experimental evidence will have to look up a large number of articles in allergological, pharmacological and other journals, and the results of each individual investigation may well be tables with numerous figures which have been subjected to a statistical analysis, but these statistical truths are not an end in themselves. They are only a means to the establishment of a coherent theory which we believe reflects the reality behind the observations. This view of science, which we have labelled *realism under empirical control,* differs markedly from that of the empiricists, like Gavaret and his successors, who hope for no more than the formulation of statistical 'laws of nature' which may serve to predict future occurrences.

Sometimes, medical scientists have such confidence in their ability to read their observations correctly that they treat biostatistics with disdain, and in order to illustrate this attitude in its extreme form, we shall quote a letter, entitled 'The present decline of medicine and its possible restoration', which was written by the endocrinologist S. G. Johnsen in the *Danish Medical Journal* [6]. He was worried that contemporary physicians are much more interested in statistical truths about groups of patients than in the individual, and he asked: 'What does it concern me that a treatment is effective in 60% of cases, if it is quite inefficient in my case?'

Being a realist, Johnsen was not particularly interested in statistical 'laws of nature', but wished to understand the underlying mechanism, and he continued in that spirit:

> The individual patient is always a surprise, and we do not really know how to tackle that problem. However, the reason for that is simply that we know much too little about the processes of the human body. If we were really able to give a complete and exhaustive description of a patient, quantitatively and qualitatively, physically and chemically, there would be no more surprises. We should know exactly the nature and extent of an active disease process, we should know exactly how the patient would fare, not only in an hour or tomorrow, but also next week or next year. It would be possible to give a precise prognosis for the individual patient and to work out a treatment plan which was correct from both theoretical and practical points of view, and the effect of the treatment would never surprise. We are very far from this goal, but we shall get there, bit by bit.

This letter was obviously meant to provoke and must not be considered a serious contribution to the philosophy of medicine, but it is worth analysing, as it reveals so well a view of medicine which has had a profound influence on medical teaching. We have already mentioned that textbook authors often deduce from biological theory 'by the laws of logic' which are the best treatments of different diseases, and we shall show later that the teaching at most medical schools is also based on the assumption that clinical medicine is little more than the application in practice of biological knowledge. We fully agree with Johnsen that progress in medicine to a large extent depends on the acquisition of more knowledge about the functions of the human body in health and disease, but we also believe that there is a great need for the empiricist approach which was first advocated by Gavaret. Johnsen, and those who agree with him, make the mistake that they do not distinguish between biological medicine, clinical medicine and clinical practice.

In order to explain what we mean by this distinction, we shall first consider a similar distinction in a different field, that between *pure science, technology* and *technique*. The physicist is a good example of someone who is concerned with pure science, and the aim of his efforts in the laboratory is to enhance our knowledge about nature. If he is also a responsible person, he will have to consider the use which others may make of that knowledge, but *qua* physicist the search for knowledge is his only objective. The technologist is also engaged in research, but his objective is a different one as he is trying to solve predefined practical problems as efficiently as possible. If, for instance, he is an aircraft engineer, he will be quite satisfied if his new model passes all the necessary tests, even though he may not be able to give a full scientific explanation of the good performance. In brief, the technologist is a seeker of *know-how*, whereas the scientist seeks to *know why*. The technician (from Greek *techne* = craft or art) is not engaged in research, but masters certain skills or techniques which enable him to carry out practical work. If the word is used in its widest sense, one may say that an aeroplane pilot is a technician.

The relationship between science and technology is complex, and it is not true to say that technology is simply applied science. The vikings who built ocean-going ships knew absolutely nothing about physics, and modern aeroplanes have to be tested in wind tunnels and in many other ways, as it is quite impossible to deduce their performance from the laws of physics. Of course, new scientific knowledge often leads to new technology, but just as often technological progress raises scientific problems.

Medicine as an academic discipline is unique, as it covers the whole range of activities. If the words are used in their original sense, one may say that members of the medical profession are engaged in science (e.g. basic research in the laboratory), technology (e.g. the testing of new drugs), and technique (e.g. examination and treatment of the individual patient). However, in ordinary language the words technology and technique suggest the development and use of complicated instruments, and we felt that it was necessary to use a different terminology in order to avoid misunderstandings. For the purpose of this discussion we have, therefore, chosen to distinguish between *medical biologists* who concern themselves with *biological medicine* (the scientific level), *clinical research workers* who are concerned with the development of *clinical medicine* (the technological level), and *medical practitioners* who are engaged in *clinical practice* (the technical level).

There can be no doubt that the theories about the circulation of the blood, the production of insulin and the aetiology of infectious diseases, as well as the 'asthma theory', belong to the level of biological medicine. The medical biologist, just like the physicist, seeks true knowledge, and his philosophical position is that of realism under empirical control, but the analogy is not complete. Physics is a pure science and, therefore, the acquisition of knowledge is the only objective, whereas all medical activities, including those on the scientific level, are subordinated to the supreme aim of medicine. Medical biologists may be engaged in basic research which has no immediate practical consequences, but they always hope that the knowledge which they acquire may some time in the future facilitate treatment or prevention of illness.

Therefore, the distinction between biological and clinical medicine is not nearly as sharp as that between physics and aircraft engineering, and the matter is further complicated by the fact that some doctors, like Johnsen, cherish the illusion that there is no real need for research on the clinical level, as they believe that it is possible—or will be possible in the future—to deduce directly from biological theory what has to be done in clinical practice.

Medical biologists rarely express their views as bluntly as Johnsen does, but exactly the same attitude is implied by the structure of the curricula at most medical schools, which is also based on the assumption that clinical practice is little more than applied biological knowledge. Students who enter medical school first study anatomy, physiology and biochemistry. Then they proceed to pathology and pharmacology, and usually they do not see their first patient until they have passed their examinations in all these biological disciplines. When the students begin their clinical training, they are, of course, taught to do a physical examination and to take a history from a patient, but at most medical centres there is no course in the general principles of clinical research. They learn little about such topics as controlled therapeutic trials, the assessment of diagnostic tests and biostatistics, and, when they leave medical school, they are unable to read critically those important papers in medical journals which recommend the introduction of new treatments and diagnostic methods. For this reason we shall take Johnsen's letter seriously, and we shall explain why we disagree and why we do not share his hopes for the future.

First of all, he underestimates the significance of biological variation. With the possible exception of monovular twins, no two human beings are ever identical, no two stomachs or pairs of kidneys are the same in all respects, and probably no two cells are exactly alike. Of course, it is also true that all human beings have many things in common and that kidneys and stomachs serve the same function in different individuals, for which reason it is possible to establish biological theories of general validity, but biological variation on all levels will forever prevent us from making exact predictions in the individual case. The physicist or chemist can be sure that any lump of pure gold will melt at 1063°C, but the prognosis of the individual patient must always remain a statistical truth. Johnsen also forgets that the course of a disease must usually be regarded as the result of a persistent interaction between the inner mechanics of the body and the environment, so that an exact prognosis requires not only extensive biological knowledge, but also full control of the stimuli from without.

Perhaps these arguments seem somewhat trivial, but unfortunately, unwarranted self-confidence on the part of biological scientists has often led to the introduction of worthless diagnostic and therapeutic methods. In the last century, Lasègue said about those of his colleagues who were particularly interested in laboratory research that 'they explain much, or rather, they explain everything, and they pass quickly from hypothesis to practice' [7], and this criticism is still justified. A few examples will be sufficient to illustrate this point.

Up to the 1950s, doctors believed that they could deduce from their theoretical knowledge that patients with chronic respiratory insufficiency ought to be given almost as much oxygen as possible, but their theoretical knowledge was incomplete, as they did not realize that oxygen treatment may cause a lethal accumulation of carbon dioxide in the blood. Excessive oxygen treatment must have shortened the lives of numerous patients.

In the 1950s and '60s, anticoagulant treatment was greatly praised as a logical and highly effective treatment of coronary thrombosis, but later clinical studies showed that the effect was minimal or non-existent.

Antibiotic treatment of gastroenteritis caused by *Salmonella typhimurium* certainly seems logical, as these microorganisms are killed by certain antimicrobial agents under laboratory conditions, but once again our theoretical knowledge is incomplete, as there is no clinical evidence that such treatment shortens the clinical course of the disease. It actually seems to prolong the period during which the bacteria are excreted in the stools.

Other treatments which proved effective have been introduced on the basis of theories which were later found to be wrong. Sulphasalazine, which is used for the treatment of ulcerative colitis, was originally introduced as an antimicrobial agent, but now it has been established that the beneficial effect is due to some other (unknown) property; alpha-methyl dopa, which is used for the treatment of hypertension, was believed to inhibit the production of noradrenalin in peripheral synapses, but now it is known to have a central effect; and the thiazides, which are also used for the treatment of hypertension, were originally believed to lower the blood pressure because of their diuretic effect, but now it is assumed that they reduce peripheral vascular resistance.

All these examples illustrate that deductions from biological theory are often unreliable and that techniques used in clinical practice must be tested empirically. Clinical practice must not be regarded as applied biological medicine, *and it is necessary to adopt the empiricist approach for the solution of clinical problems.*

Clinical research workers are of course not empiricists in the original philosophical sense, as they do not accept the ontological agnosticism (p. 17) of David Hume and the logical positivists, but they are *empiricists on the methodological level.* They fully accept that we know a lot about disease mechanisms, but they emphasize that our biological knowledge is always incomplete, that medical biologists often believe that they know more than they actually do, and that precise clinical predictions are impossible because of biological variation. Those clinicians who hold these views represent what we have called the critical clinical school, which in the 1950s and '60s revived Gavaret's ideas.

It is important to note the essential difference between realism under empirical control in biological medicine and methodological empiricism in clinical research. The medical biologist also uses statistical methods, but the end-product of his efforts is a theory—a picture of reality—which may either be true or false, whereas the end-product of clinical research is always a statistical 'law of nature' which serves to predict future events.

The controlled therapeutic trial for the comparison of two treatments is the prototype of clinical research. A consecutive series of patients are allocated at random to the two treatments and the rates of effect in the two treatment groups are compared. Such studies may be refined in a number of ways which have been discussed elsewhere [8], and in this context we only wish to make the point that the end-result of the trial is a statistical truth. The trial may, for instance, have shown that a new treatment cures 30% more patients than the current one, and perhaps the 95% confidence limits of the difference between the cure rates is 15–45% (see Chapter 7). This statistical result, which is a typical example of inductive reasoning, is what Gavaret calls 'a therapeutic law', and it serves a predictive purpose; it tells the clinician that he may expect to cure between 15 and 45% more patients, if he decides to introduce the new treatment.

In this way, clinical research workers are empiricists on the methodological level, but it must not be forgotten that the idea to do the trial may well have been some new biological theory, and in that case the result of the trial does not only provide clinical information, it also helps to test the biological theory in question. There is always a close interrelationship between research on the scientific level and research on the technological level.

Clinical research workers test diagnostic methods according to similar principles. They may, for instance, do a new test on a series of patients who are suspected of suffering from a particular disease and later calculate the rates of true positive and true negative results. Also in this case the end-result is a 'statistical truth', as it is necessary to estimate the true rates by the calculation of confidence limits. In recent years, critical clinicians have also pointed out that doctors who examine the same patient, read the same X-ray film or look at the same histological preparation do not always agree. This has been proved by inter-observer studies which reflect well the empiricist way of thinking, as the research worker does not concern himself with the objective truth of the observations, but only with the agreement between the observers.

As explained in Chapter 2, empiricism as a philosophical

position must be rejected as, clearly, it is possible to reach some insight into the workings of nature, but only the naive realist believes that our theories will ever form a completely true and exhaustive picture of reality. Therefore, Gavaret is right when he states that 'the laws of logic are insufficient for judging the effect of a new treatment' and that clinical problems must be solved by means of the law of large numbers. It is necessary to do clinical research on large numbers of patients in order to provide those numerical data—those statistical truths—which clinicians need for their predictions at the bedside.

Notes and references

1 Gotfredsen, E. *Medicinens Historie*. Copenhagen: Arnold Busck, 1950, p. 237.
2 Mason, S.F. *A History of the Sciences*. New York: Collier, 1962, pp. 220–6.
3 Fenger, C.E. Om den numeriske Methode. *Ugeskrift for Laeger*, 1839; **1**, 305–15. (Our translation from Danish.)
4 Gavaret, J. *Principes Généraux de Statistique Médicale*. Paris, 1840. (Our translation from the Danish edition, Copenhagen: Reitzel, 1840.)
5 Louis, P.C.A. *Recherches sur les Effets de la Saignée dans Quelques Maladies Inflammatoires*. Paris, 1835.
6 Johnsen, S.G. Laegevidenskabens nuvaerende forfald og mulige genrejsning. *Ugeskrift for Laeger*, 1981; **143**: 1665–6. (Our translation from Danish.)
7 Faber, K. *Nosography in Modern Internal Medicine*. London: Humphrey Milford, 1923.
8 Wulff, H.R. *Rational Diagnosis and Treatment*, 2nd edn. Oxford: Blackwell Scientific Publications, 1981.

CHAPTER 4
THE MECHANICAL MODEL

*I*n the preceding chapter it was taken for granted that medicine is a branch of natural science, and it was described how successive generations of medical scientists developed the biological theory of disease. According to that theory, disease is regarded as a fault in 'the biological machine', and, therefore, it may also be called the mechanical model.

In this chapter we shall take a much wider view of the concept of disease, and we shall criticize the biological theory. The discussion has been written as a dialogue between two medical practitioners: Dr B defends the biological theory against Dr C's critical views.

A dialogue between two philosophically minded clinicians

C: Do you accept the so-called mechanical model of disease?

B: 'The mechanical model' is just another name for the biological concept of disease, and it is usually used in a derogatory sense by those who do not like the biological approach. I am an ardent supporter of the biological approach to medical problems and, although I do not like the crudeness of the expression, I believe that in principle the mechanical model is correct. I shall try to illustrate this point of view.

I have just bought a new car and I don't think it runs as well as it ought to. I suspect that it is 'ill' and I wish to find out if my suspicion is correct. I know a mechanic well and we shall test the car. We shall measure the acceleration time from 0 to 80 mph, the idle speed of the engine, the petrol consumption and what else, and then we shall compare the results with the factory specifications for that particular model. If the car does not meet the specifications, I shall conclude that it is defective—that it functions abnormally.

This is the way doctors reason when they examine a patient. Today I saw a woman at the hospital who had moist hands and slightly prominent eyes. She complained that she was insensitive to cold, and she seemed restless. I suspected at once that she was ill and I requested a serum thyroxin and a serum tri-iodo-thyronine. If these results are abnormal, I shall conclude that I was right and that she really is ill.

The analogy is very crude, as we know much less about the mechanisms of the human body than about the workings of a motor car, but as I said before, basically it is correct. Those prescientific days have gone forever, when doctors believed in such concepts as 'the vital principle' or 'the soul'.

C: Thank you for not beating about the bush. Frankly, I do not like the idea that a human being, in principle, is no different from a motor car, but I agree that the mechanical model is part of the paradigm of contemporary somatic medicine. However, I should like you to clarify your position. You accept that the complexity of the biological mechanisms of the human body is immense and that our knowledge is limited, but let us imagine that we were able to study the structure and function of our patients' bodies in every detail. Would it then be possible to establish in each and every case, whether that particular person is healthy or ill?

B: Of course the idea is Utopian, but in principle the answer must be 'yes'. You are implying that disease is not a purely biological concept, and that the assessment of a person's health also includes value judgments. I do not accept that point of view. The question, whether or not a person is ill, is a question of fact, not a question of feelings or personal norms.

The problem of normality

C: You are—like most of our colleagues—what philosophers call a *biological reductionist*, as you reduce human beings to biological organisms and human medicine to a branch of biology. I am not at all sure that the mechanical model will stand up to a critical analysis. The first difference between your car and your patient is the obvious one that you possess a manual with the specifications for your car, whereas you do not know the specifications for your patient. What most clinicians do when they receive a laboratory report is, of course, to look up the normal range for the tests in question. They try to solve the problem of the missing specifications by resorting to the statistical concept of normality, but often they do not realize the difficulties. Traditionally, a normal range is calculated in such a way that it includes 95% of the results found in a group of normal or healthy persons, and, consequently, there is a 5% risk that a healthy person will present with an abnormal laboratory result. Then, imagine that you do ten tests on a normal person. In that case the risk that at least one of these tests is abnormal is $(1-0.95^{10})$ which amounts to 0.40 or 40%. If you do twenty-five tests (and that is not unusual in clinical practice), this chance is 72%! As Edmond A. Murphy puts it so aptly, 'Therefore, a normal person is anyone who has not been sufficiently investigated' [1].

The statistical concept of normality also raises another problem. How did the person who determined the normal range make sure that the individuals he investigated were normal or healthy? Probably, he just selected a number of individuals who felt and looked healthy, which means that the definition of health and disease according to the so-called mechanical model in the last resort depends on somebody's vague impression of the state of health of a group of people. That conclusion does not agree with your assertion that the question, whether or not a person is ill, is a question of fact and not a value judgment.

This objection is unimportant, if disease occurs so rarely that a random sample of the population for practical purposes is a sample of healthy people, but the problem is serious when disease is common. For instance, hypofunction of the thyroid gland was, at least in former days, the rule rather than the exception in some areas of the Balkan peninsula, where the iodine content of drinking water was low. A clinician who wanted to establish the normal range for serum thyroxin in such a district would not be able to equate statistical normality with health. The selection of a group of healthy people would require an independent criterion of the state of health, and no statistician can provide such a criterion. Medicine also faces similar problems today: in many developing countries malnutrition in children is the 'statistically' normal state of affairs, and in middle-aged Western European males arteriosclerosis is equally common. How do you determine the limit of normal in these cases?

B: I agree with much of that which you have been saying, but it is not right that doctors always identify normality with statistical normality. In ordinary medical usage 'normal' has two very different meanings: 'that which is common' (i.e. statistical normality) and 'that which is innocuous or compatible with health'. A double renal pelvis seen on a pyelogram may, with the same degree of justification, be labelled a harmless abnormality (abnormal = rare) and a normal variant (normal = innocuous).

Those who take the biological concept of disease—the mechanical model—seriously, are fully aware of the fact that it is unsatisfactory to equate health with statistical normality, as it invites circular arguments. Christopher Boorse, who has done much to analyse the biological concept of health, introduces the problem in this manner:

> It is a traditional axiom of medicine that health is the
> absence of disease. What is a disease? Anything which is
> inconsistent with health. If the axiom has any content a
> better answer can be given. The most fundamental problem
> in the philosophy of medicine is, I think, to break this circle
> with a substantive analysis of either health or disease [2].

In other words, the biological concept presupposes a non-statistical biological definition of normality or health, and Boorse suggests that a person is healthy if his body functions with at least species-typical efficiency, and that he suffers from disease if the functions are depressed below species-typical levels. *Disease is regarded as a deviation from the species design,* which is 'the typical hierarchy of interlocking functional systems that support the life of an organism of that kind' [3]. This idea can be applied to clinical problems. As a simple example we may imagine a person who keeps on vomiting because of a pyloric stenosis. According to Boorse, such a person is ill in the biological sense of the word, as passage from the stomach into the gut is obviously part of the species design for man. If this passage is compromised, the gastrointestinal canal does not function with species-typical efficiency and the life of the patient is endangered.

Normal function, i.e. function according to the species design, also requires that the production of thyroid hormone is kept within certain limits, as blood concentrations above or below those limits have the effect that the oxidative processes in all organs of the body are speeded up or slowed down to such an extent that their functions are compromised. Therefore, I shall say that the woman I saw at the hospital is ill, if her thyroxine is elevated, and I also maintain that the people in the Balkan mountains were ill, regardless of the frequency of a decreased thyroxine in those areas. These arguments are based on our knowledge of anatomy and physiology and not on statistical considerations.

The literature on this topic is vast, and there are others who have also tried to define either health or disease biologically. Alf Ross, independently of Boorse, concludes that a biological organism is healthy, if it functions according to the normal plan for the species [4], and J. G. Scadding has suggested the following definition of disease:

> A disease is the sum of the abnormal phenomena displayed by a group of living organisms in association with a specified common characteristic or set of characteristics by which they differ from the norm for their species in such a way as to place them at a biological disadvantage [5].

The wordings are different, but the meaning is the same: disease is a deviation from the species design, the normal plan or the norm for the species.

The threshold problem

C: You have chosen a biological yardstick for measuring your patient's state of health, but how do you distinguish between health and disease? How big must the deviation from the species design be, before you conclude that your patient is ill?

B: This is a problem, and I agree with Scadding, who concedes that the distinction between health and disease 'may require the insertion of carefully chosen, but more or less arbitrary, quantitative statements about the magnitude of deviation from the mean of normal values that will be regarded as abnormal [5]. However, as Boorse puts it: 'The precise line between health and disease is usually academic, since most diseases involve functional deficits that are unusual by any reasonable standard' [6].

C: I strongly disagree. There is very little evidence that Boorse is right on this point, and a look at the health services in Western Europe after the Second World War suggests that it is dangerous to ignore what we may call *the threshold problem*. R. E. Kendell describes the development in Great Britain: when Beveridge drew up his plans for a National Health Service 'sickness or ill health, was regarded as a fairly straightforward phenomenon, a temporary and easily recognizable departure from a natural state of health . . .' [7]. Wonderful new drugs such as penicillin and the sulphonamides had been introduced, and it seemed reasonable to assume 'that in future illnesses would, on the whole, be shorter and less severe; fewer people would die and fewer would become chronic invalids. . . . It was recognized, to be sure, that in the first few years demand on the service would be heavy. There would be a great backlog of illness that had formerly gone untreated. . . . But once this backlog had been dealt with the need for medical services would fall. . . .'

Now, we all know that this optimism was unfounded. The cost of the National Health Service nearly trebled from 1951 to 1975 (at 1950 prices) [8]; both the consultation rate in general practice and the hospital admission rate rose, and the waiting lists became longer and longer.

In Denmark the experience was the same. In 1960, 50,000 people were employed in the health service, which cost us 3.5% of the money we earned; in 1980, the number of employees had risen to 115,000, and we paid 7% of our income to the health service. During the same period, the number of hospital admissions rose by 73% and the number of doctor–patient contacts in general practice showed an annual increase of 3%.

Obviously, this growth has many aspects, but it must be admitted that it is difficult to register the beneficial effect in the available health statistics. The average expected life-span has not changed much, and hospital waiting lists have not been eliminated.

I think we must conclude that the problems are much more complex than Beveridge and his equals in other countries realized, and that the difficulties may be related to the biological concept of disease. The biological concept suggests that there is a certain *amount* of disease in a population which can be eliminated, but experience from Great Britain and Denmark seems to show that this idea is wrong. It rather looks as if the disease threshold falls when the health service expands. I agree with Kendell that 'the health service has been failing to meet the demands because, like the Norse god Thor, its staff have been trying to drink dry a vessel whose tip lies beneath the sea'.

B: You are painting a gloomy picture, but I think you miss the mark. I shall maintain that health and disease are biological concepts—just like hardness and softness are physical concepts—but I concede, as Scadding does, that the distinction between health and disease, like the distinction between hardness and softness, requires more or less arbitrary quantitative criteria.

The feeling of illness

C: I know that I have not proved as yet that 'the mechanical model' is inconsistent, but I suggest that biological reductionism of that kind has the unfortunate effect that the concepts of health and disease lose their original meaning. We must not forget that people seek medical advice because they feel ill and that the demonstration of a mechanical fault is of no importance, unless it affects the person's well-being, or serves to predict that the person's well-being will be affected some time in the future. I hold that the primary concern of clinical medicine is subjective disease and subjective health. The etymology of the words for 'illness' and 'ill' in different European languages is quite revealing, as it usually suggests subjective feelings or at least value judgments. I shall give you a few examples: *disease* in English, of course, originally meant dis-ease, and *illness* is derived from Old Norse *illr* = bad. *Pathos* in Greek means suffering, and *boljezn'* in Russian is derived from *bol'* = pain. French *maladie* is derived from *male habitus,* which means 'in a bad state', and Danish *syg* (conf. sick) originally meant worried or sorrowful. I may add that a patient (from Latin *patiens*) is one who suffers. Only the German word *krank* is compatible with the biological view. It originally meant curved or bent, suggesting that it is the purpose of medicine to straighten out the patient. That is a good example of primitive biological thinking.

We probably agree that it is the aim of medicine to eliminate disease and to preserve health, and I suggest that it is dangerous to change the meanings of these words, as it provides medicine with an aim which was not its original one. The following case history illustrates this point. A few years ago, a group of Danish cardiologists launched a campaign against untreated hypertension, and they established themselves in a number of supermarkets where they offered to measure the customers' blood pressure. A woman, who was doing her regular shopping, was found to have an elevated blood pressure, and she was referred to her general practitioner who treated her hypertension successfully. From a biological point of view everything was in order, as the woman had presented a deviation from the species design, which had now been corrected by drug treatment. However, there was one complication. Up to that day the woman had felt completely well, but now she was distressed by the fact that she had been found to be ill. Well-meaning doctors had in this case created *dis-ease* in the original sense of that word. Of course, it cannot be excluded that this woman would have suffered cardiac symptoms or a stroke some time in the future and that the antihypertensive treatment had prevented this from happening, but doctors who subscribe to a biological concept of disease may unintentionally do more harm than good. I do not suggest that doctors who support the biological view ignore their patients' subjective symptoms, but they regard them as secondary phenomena rather than necessary constituents of the concept of disease. Boorse, for instance, cannot accept the view expressed by the philosopher of medicine, H. Tristram Engelhardt, that herpes zoster is a disease 'primarily because of its pain and perhaps in part because it is somewhat unsightly'. Everyone who has had herpes zoster will undoubtedly agree with Engelhardt's statement, as this viral infection may produce very severe pain, but, as a biologist, Boorse is much more interested in the fact that the accompanying skin rash represents a deviation from the species design as regards skin function. He writes:

> ... leaving the pain aside, zoster involves two kinds of local dysfunction, neural and dermal. The skin rash alone violates the definition of normal functioning. Viewing the skin as an organ, there is no difference between failure of skin functions in a set of vesicles and failure of liver or kidney functions in local areas of those organs [9].

Perhaps it does not matter so much that we 'leave the pain aside' in a theoretical discussion, but it is unfortunate when doctors doing a wardround regard the normalization of the values on the laboratory charts as an end in itself rather than a means to alleviate symptoms and to improve the patient's quality of life.

B: Once again I think that you miss the point. I am aware of the fact that clinicians often have to make difficult value judgments and I only maintain that, on the ontological level, disease is a deviation from the biological species design. The patients' feelings are reflections of biological disturbances.

I know that there are those who identify disease with suffering, but these two concepts are not identical. The unconscious patient, and the patient with a cancer who suffers no symptoms, are in the opinion of most people seriously ill, and they *are* biologically ill, whereas the woman who suffers the pains of childbirth is considered healthy. These examples show that the use of the words 'ill' and 'healthy' in everyday language agrees well with their biological meaning.

Everybody who has tried to define health and disease in non-biological terms seems to have failed. Kräupl-Taylor, for instance, who has written a monograph on the disease concept, attempts to cut the Gordian knot by defining disease as a condition which elicits therapeutic concern. In his opinion, the indicators of morbidity are threefold:

> They are (a) a person's therapeutic concern for himself, (b) the therapeutic concern he arouses for himself in his social lay environment, and (c) the medical concern for himself he elicits in his doctor. Not every patient need have all these morbidity indicators. But every patient must have at least one of them [10].

This attempt to bypass the problems is highly unsatisfactory, as the suggested definition simply begs the question. What is it that arouses therapeutic concern? What is it that doctors treat? My simple answer is: biological disease.

The telos of life

C: I agree with the points which you have just made. As we shall discuss later, I do not wish to replace the mechanical model by a subjective concept of disease, but I am seeking a disease concept which takes into account at least both these aspects. First, however, I shall hazard the opinion that the very idea of health and disease as value-free scientific concepts is an illusion, and in order to appreciate this claim it is necessary to analyse the concept of a species design a bit further. Both Boorse and Ross [11, 12] accept that this concept has teleological overtones, as we must imagine a hierarchy of functions, each of which serves a higher-level *telos* or goal. The enzymatic processes in subcellular organelles contribute to the normal function of the cell, the cells contribute to the normal function of the organ, and the organ is important for the normal function of the individual. This train of thought obviously raises the question of the ultimate goals which seem impossible to define in scientific terms. Boorse admits that 'these highest-level goals are indeterminate and must be determined by a biologist's interests'. He writes that 'most behaviour of organisms contributes simultaneously to individual survival, individual reproduction, competence, survival of the species, survival of the genes, ecological equilibrium, and so forth', and, consequently, different biologists may use different goals as the focus of their function statements. In that case it is impossible to maintain the thesis of health and disease as value-neutral biological states.

B: I do not think that you are quite fair to Boorse. He certainly does not mean, as you suggest, that the definition of health in the last resort depends on the personal interest of the individual observer, but only that 'different subfields of biology (e.g. genetics and ecology) may use different goals as the focus of their function statements'. He continues, 'But it is only the subfield of physiology whose functions seem relevant to health. On the basis of what appears in physiology texts, I suggest that these functions are, specifically, contributions to individual survival and reproduction'.

C: I believe that we have arrived at the crucial point in this discussion. A plant biologist may accept that the goal of all the physiological processes in a plant is survival and reproduction, but even a veterinary surgeon ought to have his doubts. He may, for instance, feel that it is necessary to terminate the life of a horse or a dog in order to put an end to its suffering, and such an action implies that there is more to life, even animal life, than survival and reproduction. However, we are not here to discuss plants and animals, and I certainly do not think that the biological approach is sufficient in the case of human beings. It ignores not only the fact that members of the human species, presumably at least like other mammals, have subjective feelings; it also ignores all that which is specifically human: our self-awareness, our capacity for self-reflection and our ability to decide for ourselves what we think is important in life. The *telos* of my life is something I decide myself, and not something I read about in physiology textbooks.

I agree that biological medicine is extremely important—it constitutes the basis of most of the good things which doctors can do for their fellow human beings—but to my mind the concept of disease must include not only the biological dysfunction, but also the subjective symptoms which this dysfunction causes and the meaning which the patient assigns to those symptoms in the context of his or her own life.

Recently, I saw three patients within a short period of time who, from a biological point of view, presented almost the same problem. They all had the same 'mechanical fault', a duodenal ulcer which caused epigastric pain, and with good reason I gave them the same drug treatment. However, the meaning which these patients assigned to their illness was vastly different. The first patient had intermittently experienced duodenal ulcer symptoms for years and now took it in his stride that the ulcer had recurred; he had great confidence in the drug treatment and expected to become symptom-free within a few days. The second patient had never been ill before and feared for his life. His brother had recently died from a cancer and now he felt quite sure that he, too, suffered from a serious disease. The third patient had no great fear, but was greatly embarrassed when he was told the diagnosis. He had heard that peptic ulcers were caused by stress and he was afraid the disease might impede an expected promotion. If it became known that his work as a junior executive in a business firm had made him so stressed that he had developed a psychosomatic disease, his superiors might feel that he was not fit for a senior post.

This aspect of clinical medicine is, of course, even more important in cases of serious illness, and Eric Cassell [13] quotes the following case history as an illustration. The patient was a 35-year-old sculptress who suffered from a metastasizing carcinoma of the breast. The treatment of this mechanical fault comprised irradiation of the breast, oöphorectomy and chemotherapy, and it had been given by 'competent physicians employing advanced knowledge and technology and acting out of kindness and true concern'. Cassell discusses the problems concerning the relationship between human suffering and organic disease, and he makes the point that an understanding of the patient's suffering is not the same as knowledge of the character of the disease and the side-effects of the treatment. The pain caused by the tumour, the reduced strength of her right hand caused by the metastases in the supraclavicular lymph nodes, and side-effects like hirsutism, decreased libido, obesity, disfiguring of the irradiated breast, nausea, loss of hair, fatigue, etc., were in themselves highly unpleasant, but the source of her suffering was her interpretation of these symptoms as a self-reflecting human being in relation to her own personal situation. The illness was not only seen as a threat in terms of a greatly reduced life expectancy, but also as a threat to her integrity as a unique person shaped by a unique experience of life. She could no longer work as a sculptress and express her creative abilities, nor could she maintain the social contacts which had been the results of her artistic work. Her role as a woman was severely compromised, and she was no longer independent, but had to rely on medical competence and social assistance. According to Cassell, human suffering can only be understood if we take into account all the aspects of personhood, including, among other things, the lived past, the family's lived past, culture and society, the body, the unconscious mind and the hopes for the future.

B: You said yourself that the three duodenal ulcer patients had the same mechanical fault and that you gave them the same treatment. They simply had the same disease. Cassell's patient presented a different biological problem, a very complex one, and I can well understand her distress. However, the solution to a problem like hers is purely biological. We need to know more about the cause of cancer and we must develop more efficient treatments with fewer side-effects. Of course, I also appreciate the other problems which you mention. The fact that I regard disease as a biological dysfunction does not mean that I do not feel true concern for my patients. I agree that clinical medicine is both an art and a science, but empathic understanding of the suffering of a cancer patient can never replace the need for a thorough knowledge of the biological effects of different treatments.

C: Of course, I do not suggest that you do not feel any concern for your patients and, as I said before, scientific medicine is a tool of immense importance. In fact, doctors ought to know much more about scientific methods in order to be able to assess critically the effect of new medical technology.

However, I still strongly object to the point of view that disease and health are no more than biological concepts. We agree that normal biological function means normal biological function for a purpose, and I do not believe that the purpose or *telos* of human life can be defined in biological terms. I therefore conclude that the concepts of health and disease transgress the bounds of scientific medicine. This disagreement between us is important as all medical activity serves the preservation of health and the elimination of disease. You regard medicine as a science with humanistic overtones, whereas I believe that the science of medicine is subordinated to the art of medicine.

B: You have attacked the biological disease concept, but I notice that you have not succeeded in suggesting an alternative definition of health and disease.

C: I know. I cannot even define what is meant by a chair (see p. 4).

A comment

This discussion summarizes most of those arguments which are repeated again and again in the literature on this topic. We identify ourselves with C and, like him, we reject biological reductionism in medicine. However, that position must not be misunderstood. We accept that the mechanical model is an indispensable *part* of the disease concept and we only object to the contention that it offers a *complete* description of disease. The importance of biology is, of course, not denied as, from a realist point of view, those biological phenomena and regularities which we observe must be explained in terms of biological mechanisms, and there can be no doubt at all that the mechanical model, as part of the paradigm of modern medicine, has been extremely productive. But, as explained in the dialogue, diseases are not only biological entities. It is not biological organisms, but human beings, who are ill, and even diseases, like a duodenal ulcer or a cancer, which clearly involve a biological defect, have causes, manifestations and effects which reach far beyond the limits of biology. Therefore, clinical medicine is more than applied biology. Clinicians must also take into account their patients' experience of pain, suffering, self-respect, aim in life, etc., and they must learn to deal with such non-biological phenomena in a rational way. That is, perhaps, the biggest challenge offered by contemporary medicine. At best, the reduction of non-biological phenomena to biology is futile, and, at worst, it leads to a distorted and unacceptable view of man.

In the following chapters we shall continue our analysis of medicine as a natural science, and we shall discuss the disease classification which is based on the mechanical model. Later, we shall present what we believe is a more adequate concept of man, and we shall show that it is possible, within a wider framework of understanding, to study and discuss ethical, psychological and social phenomena in a rational way. This wider frame, which we shall characterize as *hermeneutic* (see p. 123), permits us to take into account those problems which concern values, morals and intentions, as well as those which are the concern of natural science.

Notes and references

1 Murphy, E.A. *The Logic of Medicine*. Baltimore: The Johns Hopkins University Press, 1976, p. 123.
2 Boorse, C. Health as a theoretical concept. *Philosophy of Science*, 1977; **44**: 542–73. In this very important paper Boorse defends the biological concept of

disease. We have only been able to discuss some of his arguments in this book.
3   p. 557 in [2].
4   Ross, A. Sygdomsbegrebet. (The concept of disease. In Danish.) *Bibliotek for Laeger*, 1979; **171**: 111–29.
5   Scadding, J.G. Diagnosis: the clinician and the computer. *Lancet*, 1967; ii: 877–82.
6   p. 559 in [2].
7   Kendell, R.E. The painful facts. In: Phillips, C.I. & Wolfe, J.N. (eds) *Clinical Practice and Economics*. Oxford: Pitman Medical, 1977, pp. 89–96.
8   p. vii in Phillips, C.I. & Wolfe, J.N. (eds) *Clinical Practice and Economics*. Oxford: Pitman Medical, 1977.
9   pp. 560–1 in [2]. Boorse quotes a pre-publication manuscript by H.T. Engelhardt, Jr.
10 Kräupl-Taylor, F. *The Concepts of Illness, Disease and Morbus*. Cambridge: Cambridge University Press, 1979, pp. 69–71.
11 pp. 555–6 in [2].
12 Ross, A. Det psykopatologiske sygdomsbegreb. (The psychopathological disease concept. In Danish.) *Bibliotek for Laeger*, 1980; **172**: 1–23.
13 Cassell, E. The nature of suffering and the goals of medicine. *New England Journal of Medicine*, 1982; **306**: 639–45.

CHAPTER 5
CAUSALITY IN MEDICINE

Medical thinking on all levels is pervaded by causal reasoning. Good clinicians who see a patient for the first time do not usually write a prescription straightaway, but examine the patient thoroughly. They feel that they must try to establish the cause of the symptoms before they choose the best treatment. Clinicians often express this idea by saying that they must treat the disease rather than the symptoms, and in that way they imply that the disease is the cause of the symptoms.

Medical scientists also think in terms of causality, as they seek to increase our knowledge of the causes of different diseases. They pursue this aim in different ways, as those who are engaged in laboratory research usually look for the causes inside the human body, whereas epidemiologists seek the causes in the environment.

These introductory remarks may seem somewhat trivial, but to those who are interested in medical philosophy, they invite an analysis of causation in relation to medical thinking. In this chapter we shall consider the logic of causation and the causation of disease in the individual patient, and in the next chapter we shall discuss the causal basis of the disease classification.

The logic of causation

In everyday conversation we also refer to causes and effects, and we shall approach the topic of causality by means of simple non-medical examples. The first of these concerns public telephones which are constructed in such a way that one must first insert a coin and then lift the receiver. If the telephone has been activated by the coin, a dialling tone is heard.

Telephone A is in perfect working order, as the insertion of the appropriate coin always produces a dialling tone, and as the telephone always remains dead when no coin has been put in. The insertion of the coin is a *sufficient* and *necessary* condition for activating this telephone.

Telephone B, however, is out of order. Like the first one, it is never activated when no coin has been inserted, but sometimes it also remains dead after the insertion of a coin. Therefore, the insertion of a coin is a *necessary*, but not a sufficient, condition for activating the telephone.

Telephone C is also defective, but in the opposite way. The insertion of a coin always ensures a dialling tone, but sometimes a dialling tone is also obtained when no coin has been put in. Consequently, the insertion of a coin is a *sufficient*, but not a necessary, causal factor.

This example illustrates the conventional terminology which is closely linked to the successionist or Humean view of causality (p. 19). We say that X is a necessary cause of Y, if Y is always preceded by X, and we say that X is a sufficient cause of Y, if Y always succeeds X[1].

This view of causality reflects the empiricist tradition in the philosophy of science, which was discussed in Chapter 2: if we observe again and again that two events succeed one another in a regular manner, we say that they are causally related, and we use words like *necessary* and *sufficient* to characterize the pattern of the observed sequence of events. In this way empiricists reduce causality to a psychological phenomenon; it becomes no more than an idea in the mind of the observer. Here we shall not repeat the argumentation against the empiricist position, but only point out that the empiricist view of causality has the very unfortunate consequence that statements about causal relationships must in principle be based on repeated observations. It becomes very difficult to discuss causation in the singular case.

In Chapter 2 we defended the alternative realist position in the philosophy of science, and from a realist point of view the analysis of causality in the singular case presents no problems. The realist accepts the *generative theory of causation,* and to him the statement that X causes Y means that X helps to generate Y through some mechanism or other. Causality is not an idea in the mind of the observer, but a feature of the real world which we observe. Of course, it is also from that point of view important to study the temporal relationship between the occurrence of different events, but such studies are not an end in themselves, but only a means to discover the underlying mechanism.

In order to introduce a terminology which is applicable in the singular case, we shall once again consider the three telephones. In the case of telephone C repeated observations showed that the insertion of a coin was a sufficient, but not a necessary, causal factor, but these expressions only describe the long-run experience. They do not tell us what happened at a particular time when we tried to use the telephone. If we inserted a coin and heard a dialling tone, we might well wonder whether the coin actually helped to activate the phone, or whether we might just as well have saved the coin. In other words, we might wonder whether the insertion of the coin in that particular instance was a *non-redundant* or a *redundant* factor. It was non-redundant, if it was an indispensable part of the *effective causal complex,* i.e. the sum of factors which generated the desired response, and it was redundant, if that was not the case. If we knew how the telephone worked and if we had inspected the mechanism inside the telephone at that particular time, we might have been able to answer this question.

Telephone B presented the opposite problem, as the long-run experience showed that the insertion of the coin was a necessary, but not a sufficient, causal factor. In other words, the insertion of the coin was always non-redundant, but unfortunately some other non-redundant factor was missing some of the time. Perhaps it was necessary to shake the 'phone to make it accept the coin, and whenever this was not done, it was not activated.

Telephone A presented no such problems. According to the long-run experience, the insertion of the coin was both necessary and sufficient, which means that in each instance the coin was a non-redundant factor and that in each instance no other non-redundant factor was missing.

In order to avoid terminological confusion, we shall henceforth only use the terms necessary and sufficient causal factors when we discuss *the general case,* i.e. when we refer to series of observations, whereas we shall talk about non-redundant causal factors and the effective causal complex when we refer to *the singular case*.

The next example serves to illustrate the complexity of causal mechanisms in real life. A factory burns down, and the subsequent investigation reveals at least three causal factors: (1) a short-circuit took place in one of the electrical installations, (2) a lot of inflammable material was stored nearby, and (3) the night watchman was asleep.

The example shows that it is not adequate to distinguish only between necessary and sufficient causal factors. This is of course a singular case, but, if we imagine a series of factory fires, it is obvious that these three factors were neither necessary nor sufficient. A short-circuit, for instance, is not a necessary causal factor, as factory fires may start in many other ways, and it is not sufficient, as a short-circuit is not always succeeded by a fire. The British philosopher J. L. Mackie, from whom we have borrowed this type of example, points out that this is the typical state of affairs when one tries to analyse examples from real life, and we shall show later that medicine is no exception [2].

We shall now consider the structure of the effective causal complex which led to the disaster in this particular case. This complex comprised three factors, which differed in so far as the first factor triggered, the second mediated and the third failed to prevent the course of events, but the important point is that they were all non-redundant as the elimination of any of them would have prevented the outcome. We have arrived at the important conclusion that those factors which in everyday language are said to be the causes of an event are usually neither necessary, nor sufficient, but just *non-redundant components of an effective causal complex*.

The example also shows that the delimitation of the effective causal complex is arbitrary, as one may add other non-redundant factors almost *ad libitum*. We could, for instance, include the information that the factory was partly a wooden structure, that no sprinkler system had been installed, and, if we wanted to go to the extremes, that there is oxygen in the atmosphere of the earth. We might also have included the causes of those factors which have been mentioned already, i.e. the causes of the short-circuit and the causes of the night watchman's somnolence. Usually, the list is restricted to those factors which are considered unusual under the circumstances, but we shall point out later than in medicine it is sometimes important to remember those factors which occur normally.

One does not usually ask for a long list of causes when a factory burns down. One simply asks for *the* cause of the event, and in this particular case most people would probably select the short-circuit. However, this is by no means the only possible answer, as others, with the same degree of justification, might blame the night watchman or the location of the inflammable material. In short, everyday events are determined by an effective causal complex which comprises a variety of non-redundant factors, and *the selection of 'the cause' is in the ultimate analysis the result of a choice, which reflects the interests of the person who makes the choice.* It is also worth noting that usually we only discuss the causes of undesirable events, like factory fires and the late arrival of trains. Few people would ask for the cause when a factory does not burn down or when a train arrives on time. In just the same way we are much more liable to ask for the cause of disease than for the cause of health.

The last non-medical example serves to illustrate a different type of causation. The temperature in a room is low, and there are two reasons for that: it is very cold outside and the radiators are only moderately warm. We may assume that the room temperature would become adequate, if either of these factors was eliminated (i.e. if the outside temperature rose or if we turned up the radiators), which means that we are dealing with an effective causal complex which comprises at least two non-redundant factors. Nevertheless, the example differs from the previous one, as the causal relationship is quantitative rather than qualitative, and it might even be possible to describe the relationship in terms of a mathematical function. It is a question of two *states* determining a third *state*, rather than one *event* (the short-circuit) triggering another *event* (destruction of the factory by fire). This distinction has practical consequences: our knowledge of the causal mechanism in the case of the factory fire serves a preventive purpose in so far as it may help us to prevent similar events in the future, whereas our knowledge of the causes of the low room temperature also serves a 'therapeutic' purpose. We may regulate the effect (room temperature) by manipulating one of the causal states (the radiator temperature).

Five clinical cases

In order to demonstrate the application of these ideas to clinical problems, we shall discuss five case histories. The types of problems represented by these patients are by no means rare, and the medical reader can easily find similar examples among his own patients. Such analyses serve to test one's knowledge of the causes of illness in the individual case and the rationale of the preferred treatment.

The first patient is a 23-year-old man who is admitted as an emergency, suffering from fever and neck stiffness. He is found to have meningitis and the spinal fluid contains pneumococci. Five years previously, his spleen was removed after a traffic accident, and it is known that splenectomy increases the risk of pneumococcal septicaemia and meningitis. Usually, splenectomized patients are vaccinated against pneumococci, but this was not done in this particular case.

In this case we have identified three causal factors—invasion of pneumococci, splenectomy and omission of vaccination—and the example is to a large extent analogous to that of the factory fire. If we consider a series of cases of meningitis, it will be found that these three factors are neither necessary, nor sufficient causes of that disease. Pneumococci, for instance, are not the only bacteria which generate that disease, and patients who are infected with pneumococci only rarely develop meningitis. Nevertheless, all three factors may be regarded as non-redundant components of the effective causal complex in this particular patient, and, as in the case of the factory fire, the first factor triggered, the second mediated and the third failed to forestall the outcome. However, the analogy is not complete. The introduction of the bacteria led to a *state* of infection, which manifested itself as a *state* of meningitis and, therefore, our knowledge of the disease mechanism may serve a therapeutic purpose. We may hope to cure the patient by killing the pneumococci with penicillin.

As mentioned above, doctors often talk about *the* cause of a patient's disease, and in this case most clinicians would probably say that the meningitis was caused by the pneumococci. This choice is natural from a *therapeutic* point of view, as we can eliminate this non-redundant factor, but from a *preventive* point of view it would be more reasonable to regard the omission of vaccination as the cause. The example illustrates that disease is no exception to the rule that natural phenomena always have a variety of causes; the causation of disease in the individual patient is always multifactorial, and the selection of *the* cause is the result of a choice which reflects our interests.

The second case to be discussed is a 62-year-old man with a lung cancer, who for many years had smoked 40 to 60 cigarettes a day. Most people would say that cigarette smoking was *the* cause of the cancer in this patient, and that is of course correct, as it is unlikely that the patient would have developed the cancer if he had not smoked so many cigarettes, but, on the other hand, there are numerous heavy smokers who never develop a lung cancer. In other words, the effective causal complex in this case also comprises other non-redundant factors, some of which are probably genetic.

Sometimes, doctors argue that it has been proved scientifically that, say, 70% of all cancers are caused by environmental factors, while others reply that this is not true, as it has been proved equally scientifically that, say, 85% of all cancers are genetically determined. Disagreement about such statements is, of course, absurd, as they are perfectly compatible. It is, for instance, theoretically possible that 15% of all cancers are environmentally determined in the sense that anybody develops a cancer under such environmental conditions, that 30% are genetically determined to such an extent that the persons develop their cancers regardless of the environment, and that the remaining 55% are both genetically and environmentally determined. If that is the case, it will be quite true to say that $(15+55)\% = 70\%$ of cancers are environmentally determined and that $(30+55)\% = 85\%$ are genetically determined. Some knowledge of the logic of causation may help to prevent hasty conclusions and useless discussions with political overtones.

The next two cases illustrate that it is sometimes useful to take into account non-redundant factors which are not unusual, but occur normally. A 57-year-old woman is referred to hospital because of upper abdominal pain, and the gastroscopy reveals that she has a gastric ulcer. In a case like that, one would usually conclude that the ulcer is *the* cause of the pain, but once again we are dealing with a causal factor which is neither necessary nor sufficient. It is not necessary, as patients may develop upper abdominal pain in many other ways, and it is not sufficient, as some ulcer patients have no pain. It is a non-redundant determinant of the pain in this particular patient.

The clinician decides to investigate the patient further and chooses to do a so-called pentagastrin test. He introduces a tube into the patient's stomach and finds, firstly, that her acid production is quite normal and, secondly, that there is regurgitation of bile from the duodenum into the stomach. The latter piece of information is interesting, as we know that bile regurgitation may elicit ulcer formation, but once more we have only found a non-redundant factor which is neither sufficient nor necessary. Not all patients with bile regurgitation develop an ulcer, and other factors, e.g. the ingestion of aspirin, may also cause ulcer formation.

Then, of course, the physician might study the motility of the pylorus in order to explain the regurgitation of bile, but for practical purposes it is not necessary to explore the causal network further back. The clinician will not try to treat the patient by eliminating the abnormal bile regurgitation, but he will do something quite different. As stated above, the acid production in the stomach was normal, which is quite common in gastric ulcer patients, but nevertheless the ulcer usually heals when the acid production is suppressed by drug therapy. In other words, the presence of acid in the stomach is a non-redundant determinant of the development of an ulcer, and it is possible to heal the ulcer by eliminating this normal, but non-redundant, factor. It is customary to restrict one's attention to those causal factors which represent something abnormal, but from a therapeutic point of view it is worthwhile remembering that the effective causal complex includes many non-redundant factors, both normal and abnormal, as the elimination of any of these may have a beneficial effect.

The next case illustrates the same principle. A young girl suffers from excessive menstruations and, due to the regular loss of iron, she has developed an iron-deficiency anaemia. In most such cases the doctor will not try to reduce the blood loss, as it will probably be quite sufficient to give the patient iron tablets. The patient's dietary intake of iron may have been quite normal, but the doctor may cure the patient by ensuring that the intake of iron is abnormally high.

The last example, which is more complex, but by no means unusual, illustrates some additional aspects of medical thinking.

A 44-year-old man is admitted with jaundice and ascites, and it is found that he suffers from cirrhosis of the liver. He readily admits that he has been drinking heavily for a number of years, and he explains that he drinks because of loneliness and depression. It is estimated that his daily consumption of alcohol (beer and aquavit) approaches 200 grammes. He is seen by a psychiatrist who explores the past history, and it is revealed that he had an unhappy childhood. His parents divorced when he was 5 years old and his mother had difficulties in coping with him and his two sisters. He did badly at school and was involved in petty criminality. Then, he became a carpenter and worked at building sites where it was normal to drink considerable amounts of beer during the day, but he was never employed by the same firm for more than a few years. He married young, but his wife divorced him when he started to drink heavily during long periods of unemployment. The psychiatrist also concluded from his examination that the patient had a personality disorder.

The causal complex in a case like this one is, of course, very complicated and the diagram shown in Table 2 is no more than a suggestion.

Table 2. The causal complex in a case of cirrhosis of the liver

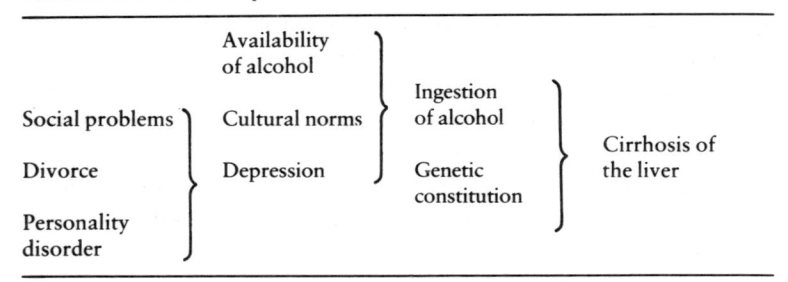

	Availability of alcohol		
Social problems	Cultural norms	Ingestion of alcohol	
Divorce	Depression	Genetic constitution	Cirrhosis of the liver
Personality disorder			

The physician who treated the patient was in no doubt that the liver disease was caused by alcoholism, as the ingestion of that amount of alcohol must be regarded as a sufficient cause of liver damage, but it is also known that the extent of the damage and the course of the disease is to some extent determined by the patient's genetic constitution.

Chapter 5

The causes of the patient's addiction to alcohol are more difficult to determine, but, according to himself, he started to drink because of his depression. However, that may not be the only non-redundant factor as he might not have become an alcoholic, if he had not belonged to a section of society where beer-drinking during the day was considered normal, and if alcoholic beverages had not been available in all grocer's shops, as they are in Denmark.

The causes of the depression are also difficult to define. The divorce had made things worse, but he had had social problems ever since his childhood, and it was also postulated by the psychiatrist that he had a character disorder, implying that his ability to tackle the problems of life might be subnormal.

At present, many people are worried about the steady rise in the number of alcoholics, and medical as well as non-medical debaters present their personal views on the matter. They sometimes believe that they know *the* cause of the problem, and, as might be expected, their choices reflect the total range of norms, interests and political beliefs in society. Some claim that alcoholism is a social disease and, in a case like this one, they might assert that the real causes were insufficient assistance to the mother, lack of individualized support at school and periods of unemployment in later life; others might prefer to blame the patient's 'weak character' which they regard as genetically determined; and yet others might stress that the patient had the wrong attitude to alcohol and that alcoholism must be fought by strict licensing laws and by teaching children the right norms. Of course, the current debate also comprises much more sophisticated points of view, but the fact remains that many discussions run astray, because the multicausality is not properly stressed.

The case history also reveals much more fundamental problems. The mechanism by which alcohol produces liver damage is not fully known, but there is no doubt that it can be explained in biological terms, i.e. in terms of morphological changes, physiological and biochemical disturbances, and immunological reactions. The first steps in the causal chain are, however, of an altogether different nature, and it is not at all clear which mechanisms are thought to be involved when social problems or mental phenomena, like a character disorder or a depression, are said to cause an increased intake of alcohol. Some psychiatrists and epidemiologists, who adopt an extreme empiricist position, simply ignore this problem and content themselves with studying the statistical correlation between psychosocial factors and the prevalence of alcoholism, while others argue that human behaviour should not be explained but understood, and that we should not explore the causes of the patient's addiction to alcohol, but try to understand his motives for starting to drink. We shall return to this extremely important topic later in this book (Chapters 10 and 14).

In this chapter we have accepted the paradigm of the mechanical model of disease, but even within that framework of reasoning we have not done full justice to the complexity of disease mechanisms. We have, for instance, ignored the influence of the defence mechanisms of the body, the mechanisms of homeostasis, and the importance of vicious circles.

It was, for instance, mentioned in connection with the first of the cases that, probably, the patient could be cured by killing the pneumococci by means of penicillin, but we ought to have added that the causation of recovery is also multifactorial. If the pneumococci are killed and the patient recovers, the effective complex which ensures this effect does not only comprise penicillin but also the action of phagocytes and antibody-producing cells. The effect of therapeutic intervention must always be viewed in connection with the *vis medicatrix naturae* [3].

In the case of the anaemic girl it was stated that the loss of iron must be replaced by an increased intake of iron, but it was not mentioned that a low iron content in the blood will have the effect that the absorption of iron from the small gut is increased and that the body by means of this *homeostatic mechanism* tries to maintain a constant iron concentration in the blood. Homeostatic mechanisms are immensely important for ensuring the steady state as regards, for instance, the concentration of hormones in the blood, the body temperature and the blood pressure.

The occurrence of *vicious circles* was demonstrated by the last clinical example, as the social problems which were said to cause the addiction to alcohol were further aggravated by the addiction.

As mentioned in the introduction to this chapter, doctors claim that they must know the cause of the patient's symptoms in order to institute rational treatment, but the discussion shows that this is a qualified truth. Usually, our knowledge of the underlying mechanisms is limited to a small number of non-redundant factors and the effect of our treatment will depend on the location of these factors in the causal network. It is this diversity which is reflected by ill-defined expressions like symptomatic treatment, curative treatment, substitution therapy and palliation, and a more stringent terminology in this area might help us to specify which effects we expect when we institute a treatment.

Notes and references

1 Sometimes it is preferable to define causal relationships *counterfactually*, which results in the following brain twisters: 'X is a *necessary* cause of Y' means 'If X had not occurred, Y would not have occurred'. 'X is a *sufficient* cause of Y' means 'If Y had not been going to occur, X would not have occurred'.
2 The presentation in this chapter is to a large extent based on J. L. Mackie's analysis of causation. The non-medical examples resemble those used by Mackie, and our 'non-redundant parts of the effective causal complex' are for all practical purposes identical with Mackie's 'inus factors' (*i*nsufficient but *n*ecessary parts of an *u*nnecessary but *s*ufficient causal complex). Mackie's theory, however, belongs to the Humean tradition, whereas we have adopted a realist view of causality. Mackie first summarized his views in the following paper: Mackie, J.L. Causes and conditions. *American Philosophical Quarterly*, 1965; 2: 245–64. The theory was later developed in great detail in: Mackie, J.L. *The Cement of the Universe. A Study of Causation*. Oxford: Oxford University Press, 1974.
3 The healing power of nature.

CHAPTER 6
THE DISEASE CLASSIFICATION: AN INDISPENSABLE TOOL

*T*here are two questions in medical philosophy which sound alike, but must not be confused: 'What is understood by disease or illness—in contrast to health?' and 'What is understood by a disease entity?'

The first of these questions, which was discussed in Chapter 4, is the concern of doctors and others alike. Illness and health are important medical terms as it is the aim of all medical activity to eliminate illness and to preserve health, but they are also important words in the ordinary vocabulary of any language, as people, even in the absence of a medical profession, would consider themselves ill or well. Some of those problems which were discussed in Chapter 4 resulted from the fact that doctors tend to define these concepts in biological or mechanistic terms, whereas the words in the ordinary language usually refer to the subjective feelings of the individual person.

The second question, which we shall discuss in this chapter, is almost exclusively a medical one. The disease classification is the tool which doctors use to pidgeonhole professional knowledge and experience, and it is to a large extent based on the mechanical model of disease. People who are not members of the medical profession may of course also use words like appendicitis and pneumonia, but the words have been borrowed from medical terminology, and they have no precise meaning except in the context of medical science.

We shall approach the analysis of the disease classification by means of a non-medical example. Imagine that somebody, who

74 Chapter 6

knows very little about the working of clocks, was asked to classify a number of defective grandfather clocks. He would probably base his classification on the type of functional disturbance and might well end up with classes like these: clocks which will not go at all even when they are wound, clocks which tick irregularly and sometimes stop, clocks which do not strike the correct number of hours, etc. A clockmaker, of course, would not accept these 'symptom diagnoses', as he would be able to pinpoint the fault in the mechanism. He would suggest 'pathogenetically' defined classes of this kind: clocks with a defective anchor escapement, clocks which are so dirty that the friction prevents normal functioning, and clocks which do not work properly due to worn notches in the locking-wheel. As a third possibility one might attempt an 'aetiological' classification and distinguish between clocks which are defective because of normal wear and tear, those which have not been looked after properly, and those which were damaged when they were moved from one place to another.

The example shows that defective clocks can be classified on different levels, and the choice of classification depends on the knowledge and interests of the observer. The clock-owner's classification only describes the problem to be solved, whereas the clockmaker's pathogenetic classification, which identifies those parts which must be repaired or replaced, clearly serves a therapeutic purpose. The third possibility, the aetiological classification, might appeal to those who are particularly interested in the preservation of old clocks, as knowledge of that kind may help to prevent functional defects.

The analogy between mechanisms of nature and the working of a clock (which of course is quite similar to the motor car analogy in Chapter 4) was used by John Locke (1632–1704) in his *Essay Concerning Human Understanding* which we shall quote several times in this chapter. Locke is a realist as he believes that our perceptions of natural phenomena, like the manifestations of disease, are caused by the mechanisms and structures—the real essence—of the things perceived, but he also believes that the perceiver has no knowledge of this real essence. He writes that our perceptions or ideas are

> ... more remote from the true internal constitution from which these qualities flow, than ... a countryman's *idea* is

from the inward contrivance of that famous clock at Strasburg, whereof he only sees the outward figure and motions. . . . Therefore we in vain pretend to rank things in sorts, and dispose them into certain classes, under names, by their *real essences,* that are so far from our discovery or comprehension [1].

Locke's disbelief in our ability to apprehend the sources of our perceptions was undoubtedly justified in the late 17th century, but, as explained in the previous chapters, it would be an expression of undue scepticism to maintain today that we possess no knowledge of the structure and functions of the clockworks of nature. Our knowledge of biological mechanisms may still be limited, but we are often able to pinpoint some of the factors which cause human illness, and the present disease classification is to a large extent based on this incomplete knowledge. We wish to discuss this important point in some detail and, with that purpose in mind, we shall give a brief account of the gradual development of the disease classification during the last two centuries.

The history of the classification of diseases

Until the end of the 18th century, doctors, observing their patients and listening to their complaints, could well be likened to a countryman studying the clock in Strasbourg, as they could only classify their patients according to the clinical pictures. They made diagnoses like dropsy, phthisis (wasting), diabetes (running through), typhus (stupor) and variola (mottled appearance), and some enthusiastic taxonomists, like Linnaeus and Sauvages, even believed that it was possible to distinguish between genera and species of disease in the same way as they distinguished between genera and species of plants and animals (p. 34). Even today, the disease classification comprises many clinical syndromes which can only be defined by the patients' clinical pictures, as we still know next to nothing about the underlying mechanisms.

It was also mentioned in Chapter 3 that doctors at the beginning of the 19th century began to do routine autopsies and gradually got used to identifying diseases with anatomical lesions. This was a completely novel idea which had a tremendous impact on medicine, and even today the majority of disease names are borrowed from the terminology of morbid anatomy (e.g. gastric ulcer, myocardial infarction and cholecystitis). In order to illustrate what happened, we may imagine that doctors at that time observed a number of patients with upper abdominal pain, and that they found that some of these had a gastric ulcer. As explained on page 67, the ulcer is neither a necessary nor a sufficient cause of upper abdominal pain, but due to their preoccupation with morbid anatomy, doctors focused their attention on this particular finding. The gastric ulcer is no more than a non-redundant causal factor in some patients with upper abdominal pain, but now it was bestowed the status of a disease entity, and doctors wrote textbook chapters on *gastric ulcer disease*, in which they discussed its causes and manifestations.

A few decades later, doctors developed an interest in human physiology, and it is as though they had acquired a new kind of spectacles which made them see physiological disturbances where before they had only seen anatomical lesions. This new mode of thought also had a profound effect on the disease classification, and for a while, patients with upper abdominal pain who had previously been said to suffer from gastric or duodenal ulcers, were said to suffer from hypochylia or hyperchylia, i.e. decreased or increased production of gastric juice. These particular diagnoses were quickly abandoned and once again replaced by the old anatomical ones, but many other physiologically defined disease entities are still accepted. Graves' disease was redefined as hyperthyroidism (hyperfunction of the thyroid gland) and diabetes mellitus was recognized as a disturbance in carbohydrate metabolism. The interest in physiology also led to the establishment of new disease entities. At the turn of the century, for instance, the invention of the sphygmomanometer led to the discovery that some patients, as part of the pathogenetic causal network, had a high blood pressure, and *arterial hypertension* became a recognized diagnosis.

During the second half of the last century, the foundation was also laid to modern microbiology, and patients with infectious diseases were reclassified according to the species of the infective agent. For example, it had previously been recognized that some patients suffering from the clinical syndrome, phthisis, presented certain anatomical lesions, tubercles, and the anatomically defined disease entity, tuberculosis, had been established. Now, however, the infective agent was discovered and tuberculosis was redefined as illness caused by *mycobacterium tuberculosis.* This was a very important phase in the history of the disease classification for two reasons. Firstly, it became possible for the first time to define a large number of disease entities aetiologically and, secondly, the dogma of unicausality (one cause—one disease) was further established. As pointed out in the preceding chapter, this dogma is also fallacious in the case of most infectious diseases, as the bacterium or virus must usually be regarded as one of many non-redundant causal factors in the individual patient.

The disease classification is still largely a mixture of disease entities defined in anatomical, physiological and microbiological terms, but it continues to develop. During recent years, medical scientists have taken a great interest in immunology, and immunologically defined disease entities are being established [2].

The status of a disease entity

This ultrashort exposition of the history of the classification of disease stresses the point that it is a man-made classification of individual patients. Doctors have studied millions of sick people, and we must imagine that no two of these were ever completely identical as regards their clinical pictures and the underlying causal mechanisms, but in order to build up a medical science, it was essential to stress the similarities rather than the differences. It was necessary to establish a classification of patients in order to classify clinical knowledge and experience. According to this point of view, there are no genera and species of disease, and disease names may be regarded as labels which we attach to groups of patients which resemble each other in those respects which we consider important. Locke expresses the idea in general terms in the following passage:

> To conclude . . . all the great business of *genera* and *species,* and the *essences,* amounts to no more than this, that men making abstract *ideas,* and settling them in their *minds,* with names attached to them, do thereby enable themselves to consider things, and discourse of them, as it were in bundles, for the easier and readier improvement, and communication of their knowledge, which would advance but slowly, were their words and thoughts confined only to particulars [3].

In philosophical terminology this position is usually called *nominalistic*, as a universal (e.g. a disease or a zoological species) is regarded as a name (*nomen*) which is attached to a bundle of particulars, and in medicine the idea has been concisely expressed by the following dictum, which is attributed to Rousseau: Il n'y a pas de maladies, il n'y a que de malades (there are no diseases, only sick people).

However, the Lockean version of nominalism also stresses the point that our classifications of natural phenomena are not arbitrary, as they must be moulded on the realities of nature. Locke also writes:

> I would not here be thought to forget, much less to deny, that nature in the production of things, makes several of them alike: there is nothing more obvious, especially in the races of animals, and all things propagated by seed. But yet, I think, we may say, the sorting of them under names, *is the workmanship of the understanding, taking occasion from the similitude* it observes amongst them, to make abstract general ideas ... [4].

He continues:

> For though men may make what complex *ideas* they please, and give what names to them they will; yet if they will be understood, when they speak of things really existing, they must, in some degree, conform their *ideas* to the things they would speak of ... [5].

In other words, the domestic cat or *Felis domesticus*, as a species, is an idea produced by the human mind, but it is based on the existence in nature of a group of animals which resemble each other more closely than they resemble animals which are referred to other species. They resemble one another as regards both their appearance and their genetic constitution (which in Locke's terminology must be regarded as part of the real essence), and one may say that they constitute a natural *kind* and not just an arbitrary *set* of animals.

Medical writers, ever since the days of Linnaeus and Sauvages, have emphasized the analogy between the disease classification and the taxonomies of zoology and botany, and in the case of some disease entities this is easy to understand. Patients with measles, for instance, distinguish themselves from patients with all other diseases to such an extent that the diagnosis in the vast majority of cases is obvious to any experienced physician. The clinical course varies little from patient to patient, the rash is highly characteristic, and medical science has shown that patients with this disease do not only constitute a natural kind on the *clinical level,* but also on the *pathogenetic* and the *aetiological* levels. In all cases the measles virus is a non-redundant aetiological factor, and the spread of the virus through the body—the pathogenesis—presents little variation [6].

Measles, however, is the exception rather than the rule. The disease entity tuberculosis is, like measles, aetiologically defined, and patients suffering from this disease also resemble each other in other respects: the affected organs contain tubercles which have a characteristic appearance under the microscope, the course of the disease in untreated patients is often one of slow progression, and the patients respond to those drugs which kill the bacteria. However, unlike measles, patients with tuberculosis present a great variety of clinical pictures, and it is not possible to diagnose the disease without the use of paraclinical methods of investigation. Clinically, some patients can hardly be distinguished from patients with cancer of the lung, while others are indistinguishable from patients with certain chronic diseases in the gut or the spine. Therefore, tuberculosis constitutes a natural kind on the *aetiological* level, but not on the *clinical* level.

Most diseases in the current classification are defined *pathogenetically,* and, as an example, we may consider diabetes mellitus. This disease entity is today defined by a decreased ability to metabolize ingested glucose, and it is a useful diagnosis as the patients require the same type of diet and to some extent respond to the same treatments. However, patients with diabetes also present a variety of clinical pictures and they differ greatly as regards the causal mechanisms which produce the functional disturbance. In some the pancreas produces too little insulin and in others the responsiveness to insulin seems to be decreased. Diabetes mellitus (from *diabaino* = pass through, and *mellitus* = sweet) was originally defined clinically by the ample discharge of sweet urine, but since its redefinition as a functional disturbance it no longer represents one natural kind on the clinical level.

We may summarize these arguments as follows: centuries ago, doctors began to classify patients according to their directly observable clinical characteristics. They found that some patients resembled each other in a number of aspects and each such 'natural kind' constituted a clinical syndrome. As we shall discuss below, such syndromes were never well defined, but the authors of medical textbooks described 'the typical cases' of each disease, and then clinicians could diagnose these diseases when their patients resembled the typical cases. The purpose, of course, was inductive, as clinicians expected that their patients, within limits, would have the same prognosis and respond to the same treatments as the standard cases in the textbooks. Later, these clinical diagnoses were replaced by others which were defined on the pathogenetic or aetiological levels as it was found that these new entities permitted much more precise predictions and facilitated the development of specific treatments. However, the new disease entities were less homogeneous on the clinical level, for which reason the development also required the introduction of a multitude of refined diagnostic methods.

According to W. V. Quine (b. 1908), this process is typical of the development of a science. He believes that man has an innate ability to recognize natural kinds, as illustrated by the fact that even primitive man, searching for food, must be able to classify objects according to, for instance, colour, shape and smell. This ability is also of fundamental importance to scientists, but the sophisticated nature of their activities requires that they learn to recognize qualities which are not directly observable. Quine writes:

> Credit is due to man's inveterate ingenuity, or human sapience, for having worked around the blinding dazzle of color vision and found the more significant regularities elsewhere.... He has risen above it by developing modified systems of kinds, hence modified similarity standards for scientific purposes. By the trial-and-error process of theorizing he has regrouped things into new kinds which prove to lend themselves to many inductions better than the old [7].

In order to demonstrate the difference between diseases defined on the clinical, pathogenetic and aetiological levels, we have compared the disease classification with the classification of defective clocks and, like many others, we have also compared it with the taxonomies of animals and plants, but unfortunately these analogies are equally imperfect.

First of all, neither analogy pays due respect to the dynamic character of disease processes. The pathologist may describe the lesions in the heart in *rheumatic heart disease,* but clinicians making this diagnosis have in mind, not only the morphological changes of the mitral valve, but also the course of the disease process: they imagine that the patient once had a streptococcal throat infection which elicited an immunological reaction—which led to an endocarditis—which again led to slowly progressing scarring of the heart valves—which explains the observed signs of cardiac failure. The natural kinds which we try to recognize are not kinds of disease states but kinds of disease processes. Further, these disease processes do not take place in relatively closed systems, like the case of the grandfather clock in the dining room, but in a human body which perpetually interacts with the environment. The prognosis of endocarditis in post-streptococcal rheumatic fever varies, and one of the factors which determine the outcome may well be the patient's environmental conditions. Clinicians sometimes talk about the *natural history* of a disease, as if it was programmed from the start to run a certain course, but this concept is little more than a myth.

The analogy between zoological taxonomy and the disease classification is also rendered imperfect by the fact that the zoologist attempts to establish an exclusive and exhaustive classification, whereas the medical taxonomist cannot hope to achieve this end. The disease classification is not an exhaustive classification of patients, as many patients cannot be classified in one of the recognized disease entities; nor is it an exclusive classification, as the same patient is often said to suffer from several diseases which may either be unrelated (like influenza in a patient with hypertension) or related, reflecting different aspects of the same disease process (like bronchial asthma and emphysema).

Diseases as demons or divine ideas

We hope that these views of the structure of the disease classification are acceptable to the reader. They reflect the historical development of the classification and, philosophically, they fit in with Locke's version of nominalism. However, if our views are acceptable, it is not because doctors usually think along these lines. Anybody who has listened to conversations between members of the medical profession will have heard numerous statements of this kind: 'Duodenal ulcer disease usually attacks men'; 'Crohn's disease may manifest itself in different ways'; 'This disease was only discovered a few years ago'; and 'This patient suffers from arterial hypertension'. Expressions of this kind, which are part of medical idiom to such an extent that we have not even been able to avoid them completely in this presentation, reflect a very different attitude to the status of a disease entity. They are incompatible with the nominalist view that the disease classification is man-made, but suggest that diseases are 'things' which exist in themselves and which are *discovered* by doctors. Diseases are regarded almost as demons which *attack* people and cause *suffering* by *manifesting* themselves in the persons they have attacked. It is interesting that this alternative view of the status of a disease entity is not only heard in informal conversations, but is also found in sophisticated analyses of clinical thinking. Alvan Feinstein, for instance, writes in his book *Clinical Judgment* that illness in the individual patient is the result of an interaction between a disease and a host [8].

Such formulations bring to mind Plato's philosophy. It may be remembered that Plato regarded universals as divine ideas, which were real, eternal and unchangeable, whereas particulars were no more than transitory reflections of these ideas. According to that view, the idea of *Felis domesticus* is real and eternal, and all the individual cats which we see around us are just imperfect copies of the idea. The mysterious disease, which in Feinstein's book interacts with a host, may be interpreted along these lines: it represents the Platonic idea, whereas the illness of the individual patient is the imperfect reflection of the idea. The typical cases which are described by the authors of medical textbooks may also be likened to Platonic ideas, which are copied, often rather unsuccessfully, by the patients seen by the clinician on his wardround.

Of course, we do not wish to imply that any doctor believes that diseases are demons which attack people, or that doctors subscribe to the doctrines of Plato's philosophy, but, nevertheless, they tend to overlook that the disease classification is man-made and they assume unreflectingly that disease entities somehow have an independent existence. We believe that this attitude to the disease classification, which we shall label the *Platonist attitude,* has a number of subtle consequences.

Consequences of the Platonist view

The unreflecting Platonist takes the disease classification for granted and it does not pass his mind to ask himself whether it could be improved and to what extent it serves different purposes. If, however, we stop to consider the structure of the classification, it is immediately obvious that it is much better suited to hospital practice than to general practice. It requires chemical blood analyses, X-ray examinations and sometimes highly specialized investigations to demonstrate the abnormalities which define the disease entities, and the general practitioner who is unable to perform or request all these investigations, or believes that they are unwarranted in the majority of his patients, is often scorned by his hospital colleagues for not finding out what is *really* the matter with his patients. Some general practitioners, like Krogh-Jensen [9], have tried to tackle this problem by suggesting an alternative standardized classification suitable for general practice, and such classifications might help the general practitioner to predict more accurately which patients will recover without therapy, which patients require special treatments and which patients must be referred to hospital for further investigations.

The Platonists among doctors are also likely to miss the point that the disease classification serves a therapeutic rather than a preventive purpose. It is often said that the health services must divert a greater part of their resources to prevention, but it is not usually appreciated that the development of preventive medicine is hampered by the structure of the disease classification. Traditionally, most diseases are defined pathogenetically 'by the defective cogwheel' and interference at that level only serves to repair the damage. The diagnosis of hyperthyroidism tells us to give anti-thyroid drugs, the diagnosis of a cancer of the colon suggests surgical removal, and the diagnosis of vitamin B_{12}-deficiency anaemia invites treatment with vitamin B_{12}, but these diagnoses suggest no preventive measures, as we know next to nothing about the aetiological causal factors (environmental or genetic factors) which elicit the disease processes. In general, one must imagine that the complex of aetiological factors which starts off the disease process differs greatly from patient to patient, and those who hope to be able to prevent pathogenetically defined diseases by some single measure are apt to be disappointed. Epidemiologists, for instance, have done their very best to explore the complex aetiology of myocardial infarction, but they always end up by finding a number of so-called risk factors which may well be statistically significant, but do not enable us to prevent the disease with any degree of certainty in the individual person. Possibly, intervention trials which eliminate a number of risk factors will show some effect, but, generally speaking, we may be attacking the problem in the wrong way. Perhaps we should not spend quite so much time and effort trying to explore the causal network backwards from effect to causes—from an anatomical lesion to the multiple aetiological factors—as it might prove much more profitable to do prospective studies of the effects of different aetiological factors and to reason from cause to effects. We might, for instance, follow cohorts of people who are exposed to certain chemicals, who work in certain industries, who are unemployed, or who are living under career pressure, and we might find that one aetiological factor contributes to a lot of illness which does not fit the therapeutically orientated disease classification. We know, for instance, that cigarette smoking promotes the development of a variety of diseases, including lung cancer, chronic bronchitis, acute myocardial infarction and cancer of the bladder. Doctors who are especially concerned with preventive medicine might attempt to establish their own aetiological disease classification which would include entities like cigarette disease, alcohol disease, organic solvent disease as well as many others which are still unrecognized. This idea is, of course, by no means new, as illustrated by disease entities like hatter's shakes, farmer's lungs, pidgeon breeder's disease and the KZ-syndrome (i.e. the late effects of imprisonment in concentration camps).

Infectious diseases differ from most other disease entities as they may be regarded as both aetiologically and pathogenetically defined. The microorganism may be regarded as an aetiological factor as it represents the external cause of the disease, but it may also be regarded as a pathogenetic factor, as it produces the disease inside the body. Therefore, microbiologically defined diseases are ideal for both preventive and therapeutic purposes.

The world of ideas in Plato's philosophy is a static one, and it may well be one of the consequences of a Platonist attitude that doctors tend to underestimate the temporal and geographical variation of the spectrum of illness. One of the authors of this book first developed an interest in the structure of the disease classification when, as a Danish medical student, he visited a Yugoslav Hospital in the 1950s. He had learnt to accept that the patients at the teaching hospital in Copenhagen did not always resemble the 'typical' cases in the textbooks, and he only became aware of this problem when he saw the patients in the wards at the university hospital in Sarajevo. The Bosnian patients resembled the patients in the Danish textbook much more closely than contemporary Danish patients. They had 'typical' rheumatic fever, they developed the 'typical' complications of pneumonia and they suffered from tuberculous spondylitis and other diseases which were described in the textbook, but were rarely seen at home. The explanation was, of course, that the textbook described those patients who had been seen in Danish hospitals decades earlier. Textbook authors tend to forget that the classification and description of diseases must fit the spectrum of illness in a particular cultural setting at a particular time, and there is little doubt that the spectrum changes. As a single example, gastric ulcer disease in the 1880s usually 'attacked' young women and led to many acute complications, whereas today it is mostly a disease of elderly men and women [10]. Geographical variation is also prominent, and it is a major problem of medical education that many medical students all over the world read American and British textbooks which do not describe the patients in their own countries.

The next problem to be discussed is the lack of explicit definitions of those diseases which are described in medical textbooks, and we shall approach this topic by means of a rather unrealistic non-medical example. Imagine that we wished to explain the meaning of the word *chair* to somebody who belonged to a culture where this kind of object was completely unknown. Probably, we should not bother to formulate a formal definition as it would be much easier simply to show the visitor a few typical chairs and to explain their function. By referring to these standards he would gradually learn to use the word correctly, and he would find, as we do, that it does not hamper communication to any significant extent that the demarcation of this kind of object is somewhat fuzzy and that there is a gradual transition between chairs, stools and similar pieces of furniture (cf. p. 4).

Medical students learn to recognize different diseases in exactly the same way, as textbook authors and clinical tutors do not attempt to define different diseases but confine themselves to the description and demonstration of typical cases. These cases, which may be likened to Platonic ideas, serve as useful standards of reference, but the procedure does not take into account that the fuzziness, which was acceptable in everyday conversation as regards chairs, poses a major problem in clinical medicine. If two persons were asked to point out the chairs among all the other objects in a private home, there would undoubtedly be close agreement, but if two clinicians are asked to diagnose the patients in the same medical ward, there is bound to be considerable disagreement. There are several reasons for this.

In some cases there is a gradual transition between disease and normality or between two diseases, and the number of borderline cases may be so large that clinical research workers who use slightly different criteria may obtain very different results. For instance, the recorded prognosis of hypertension to a large extent reflects the definition of a normal blood pressure, and the reported results of surgical treatment of duodenal ulcers depend on the in- and exclusion of praepyloric ulcers. Problems of this kind can only be solved by arbitrary demarcation of the disease entities. To quote Locke: 'the boundaries of species are as man, and not as nature makes them' [11].

In other cases the presence or absence of an anatomical lesion which defines a disease entity cannot be established with certainty when a patient survives. It will, for example, be explained in the next chapter that the diagnosis of acute myocardial infarction is often based on indirect evidence, and two clinical observers may well disagree on the diagnosis in the individual case. This particular problem could be solved by establishing clinical working definitions, which would ensure that at least clinical research workers base their diagnoses on similar criteria.

However, those disease entities which present the biggest problem are clinical syndromes, like, for instance, systemic lupus erythematosus and the other connective tissue diseases. In such cases the diagnosis rests on a total evaluation of the clinical picture and it is up to the individual clinician to decide whether his patient resembles the typical textbook case to such an extent that the diagnosis is warranted. The present state of affairs is well illustrated by the chapter on systemic lupus erythematosus in Harrison's well-known *Principles of Internal Medicine* [12]. The authors propose no definition of systemic lupus, but nevertheless they state that 92% of patients with this disease suffer from arthritis or arthralgia, that 61% have leucopenia, and that 'abundant evidence indicates that appropriate treatment may suppress flare-ups and prolong life'. The authors have forgotten Rousseau's dictum that 'there are no diseases but only sick people' and the information which they provide is of limited value when they do not tell us which patients they are writing about.

The disease classification is an indispensable tool in clinical medicine, but due to the lack of explicit clinical definitions, the recording of clinical experience is at present much too imprecise. Doctors have treated thousands of patients who were said to suffer from systemic lupus erythematosus and, if the disease had been clearly defined, it would have been possible to state the prognosis in exact probabilistic terms. Now, however, the collective experience is so imprecise that even the authors of Harrison's textbook can only write that appropriate treatment has some effect, and this example is by no means exceptional.

There is a great need for generally accepted working definitions of clinical syndromes, but, taking a longer view, we must also hope that one day we shall know so much about those mechanisms which generate the observed symptoms and signs that it will prove possible to redefine such disease entities. In general, knowledge of the 'real essence' permits more stable definitions which depend less on convention.

The philosophical problem which underlies the discussion in this chapter is the age-old dispute about universals, and we have tried to navigate between the Scylla of essentialism (or Platonism) and the Charybdis of extreme nominalism. Essentialism underlines correctly that any classification of natural phenomena must reflect the realities of nature, but it ignores the fact that classifications also depend on our choice of criteria and that this choice reflects our practical interests and the extent of our knowledge. Nominalism, on the other hand, stresses correctly the human factor, but the extreme nominalist overlooks that classifications are not arbitrary but must be moulded on reality as it is. Locke was one of the first philosophers who saw this conflict clearly, and we believe that his theory which combines both views is particularly well suited for the analysis of the disease classification. We also hope to have shown some of the practical consequences of this ancient philosophical conflict.

Notes and references

1 Locke, J. *An Essay Concerning Human Understanding* (originally published 1690) ed. P.H. Nidditch. Oxford: Oxford University Press, 1975, Book III, Chapter VI, § 9, p. 444.
2 The first immunologically defined disease which has become well known to the general public, is AIDS (acquired immunodeficiency syndrome). It was first described in young homosexuals who had developed a particular malignant tumour (Kaposi's sarcoma), and it is now known that the patients are infected with a particular virus. However, those who named the syndrome focused neither on the aetiology nor on the anatomical lesion, but on the immunological causal factor.
3 p. 420 (Book III, Chapter III, § 20) in [1].
4 p. 415 (Book III, Chapter III, § 13) in [1].
5 p. 456 (Book III, Chapter VI, § 28) in [1].
6 In this discussion we distinguish between natural kinds on the clinical, pathogenetic and aetiological levels. A natural kind on the clinical level is a class of patients which is defined by a regularly occurring constellation of symptoms and signs. Such a class does not constitute a natural species in the Lockean sense, as it is defined by its nominal essence, and not by its real essence, but it resembles the natural kinds of Quine's theory. See [7].
7 Quine, W.V. *Ontological Relativity and Other Essays* (Chapter 5, Natural kinds). New York: Columbia University Press, 1969, p. 128.
8 Feinstein, A.R. *Clinical Judgment.* Baltimore: Williams & Wilkins, 1967, p. 25.
9 Krogh-Jensen, P. *Praksis sygdomsklassifikation.* (Disease classification in general practice. In Danish.) Copenhagen: Laegeforeningens forlag, 1976.
10 Wulff, H.R. *Rational Diagnosis and Treatment*, 2nd edn. Oxford: Blackwell Scientific Publications, 1981, pp. 62–3.
11 p. 457 (Book III, Chapter VI, § 30) in [1].
12 Mannik, M. & Gilliland, B.C. Systemic lupus erythematosus. In: Harrison's *Principles of Internal Medicine*, 10th edn. New York: McGraw-Hill, 1983, pp. 387–91.

CHAPTER 7
PROBABILITY AND BELIEF

*P*robability is a key concept in clinical thinking. No clinician who returns home from a busy day in his practice or at a hospital is spared the uncomfortable feeling that some of his diagnoses may prove to be wrong and that some of his treatments may not have the desired effect. Much too often he has encountered the unexpected, and he has learnt to accept that diagnostic and prognostic assessments are rarely certain, but more often *probable* to a varying degree.

The clinician feels the same when he is reading his medical journals. Every week he is confronted with new scientific results, but experience has taught him that the well-established facts of today may be refuted in some other medical journal the following week. When he reads that some new treatment is superior to the ones he is using already, he will assess the evidence critically, and at best he will conclude that *probably* it is true.

In this chapter we shall explore the notion of probability and hope in that way to approach some of the basic problems of medical thinking.

Two concepts of probability

The statistical probability concept is so widely accepted that any school child who studies mathematics is indoctrinated with the idea that a probability is a *frequency*. It is not, of course, an ordinary frequency which can be determined by simple observation, but it is the *ideal* or *true* frequency, which underlies the observed frequency.

Imagine, for instance, that we possess a die which looks somewhat asymmetric, and that we wish to determine the probability of obtaining sixes. To solve this problem we shall rely on the *law of large numbers*, which means that we shall throw the die a large number of times as we know that in the long run the observed frequency will approach the true probability. Statisticians often use the expression that a probability is a long-run frequency, and a probability which is defined in this way will in this chapter be called *a frequential probability*.

The exact magnitude of a frequential probability will always remain unknown, as we cannot make an infinite number of observations, but, when we have made a series of observations, the statistician can calculate the so-called confidence interval which is likely to include the true, frequential probability. Imagine, for instance, that we have thrown the die 200 times and that we obtained twenty sixes. In that case, the observed frequency of sixes is 10%, and the statistician will tell us that the 95% *confidence interval* is 6–15%, which means that we can be fairly certain that the probability lies within this interval [1]. We cannot be absolutely certain that this is the case, but the statistician will assure us that in 95% of cases such a confidence interval includes the probability, i.e. the true frequency.

The width of the confidence interval depends on the number of observations. Imagine that somebody selects fifty Danes at random and finds that forty of them have blond hair. Then, the observed frequency of blond hair is 80%, and the statistical calculation will show that the 95% confidence interval is 66–90%. Consequently, the observer may feel fairly confident that the true frequency of blond Danes is above 66% and below 90%. If, instead, 500 Danes are selected and 400 are found to have blond hair, the observed frequency is still 80%, but the calculated 95% confidence interval is 76–83%. In that case, he may feel fairly certain that the true frequency is above 76% and below 83%. Medical research workers often base their conclusions on studies of a limited number of patients and, as we shall discuss below, the calculation of confidence limits is an important aid when clinicians wish to make probabilistic statements on the basis of their experience.

The frequential probability concept is so widely accepted that we tend to forget that words like probability, chance, risk and odds, are also used in the ordinary language in a very different sense. Imagine, for instance, that somebody says 'that N.N. will probably come on Tuesday'. This statement simply implies that the person who made the statement *believes* or *expects* that N.N. will turn up, and it provides no information as regards the basis of this expectation or belief. According to the *Shorter Oxford English Dictionary*, something may be regarded as a probability, if it is 'something which, judged by present evidence, is likely to be true, to exist, to happen', and the nature of that evidence may vary from case to case. In this particular instance it is, of course, possible that the person who made the statement has observed that N.N. usually turns up on Tuesdays, but it is also possible that it never happened before: the person may simply feel that he knows N.N. so well that he can predict that N.N. will make up his mind to come this time.

A probabilistic statement always implies some degree of uncertainty, and, as illustrated by the following examples, one may quantify the degree of one's belief in the occurrence of a particular event: before the launching of the first space-shuttle, a critical TV-commentator said that there was only a *95% probability* that it would return safely from its maiden trip; a politician once told his friends that there was a *fifty-fifty chance* that he would win the election; and a gambler stated that the *odds* against a certain horse were four to one, meaning that there was a 20% probability that it would win.

Superficially, such probabilities look like frequential ones, but a close look at the statements will show that this is not the case. We are concerned with unique events—the maiden trip of the space-shuttle, that particular election and that particular race—and it simply makes no sense to apply the statistical idea that a probability is a long-run frequency. The space-shuttle, for instance, will either return or not return, and it makes no sense to say that in the long run the frequency of safe returns from the maiden trip is 95%. In principle, there is no difference between these statements and the statement 'that N.N. will probably come on Tuesday', apart from the fact that in these cases an attempt has been made to quantify the magnitude of the belief in the occurrence of the event. In order to explain the meaning of such quasi-frequential statements, one may say that the TV-commentator's belief in the safe return of the space-shuttle was the same as his belief in picking a red marble from a bag containing ninety-five red and five white marbles, and that the gambler's belief in the victory of that particular horse was the same as his belief in picking a red marble from a bag containing twenty red and eighty white marbles.

In conclusion, we have at our disposal two probability concepts, which must not be confused. In *statistics*, a probability is the ideal or true frequency which underlies an observed frequency, and such probabilities are called frequential probabilities. In the ordinary language, a probability is a measure of our subjective belief in the occurrence of a particular event (or, as we shall explain later, in the truth of a hypothesis). Such probabilities, which may be quantified so that they look like frequential ones, are called subjective probabilities [2].

We shall now apply these ideas to two diagnostic problems.

Two clinical examples

A man seeks medical advice because of praecordial pain. The electrocardiogram presents an abnormal pattern and the aminotransferase concentration is slightly elevated. A cardiologist who sees the patient concludes that there is a 90% probability that this patient suffers from acute myocardial infarction.

Let us imagine that we ask the cardiologist what he means by this probabilistic statement. He cannot very well argue that he knows from experience that 90% of such patients suffer from myocardial infarction, because most patients who are suspected of this disease survive, and in all such cases one can never know for sure whether the diagnosis was correct. The cardiologist will, of course, have seen some patients who died and who were found to have an infarction at autopsy, but he cannot extrapolate his experience from those patients who died to those who survive, as it may be argued that those who died did so because they had an infarction. Consequently, the statement is not based on an observed frequency.

Instead, the cardiologist bases his probabilistic statement on his knowledge of pathophysiology. Interruption of the blood flow through one of the coronary arteries produces myocardial damage, and the aminotransferase which is usually contained within the muscle cells leaks into the blood stream. At the same time, the conduction of electric impulses through the heart is disturbed and electrocardiographic changes, like those seen in this patient, appear. From this knowledge, which is based on both human studies and animal experiments, the cardiologist concludes that his belief in the diagnosis of acute myocardial infarction in that particular patient is as strong as his belief in picking a red marble from a bag containing ten white and ninety red marbles. The probability in this case was definitely a subjective probability.

Then consider this example: *A female patient who suffers from abdominal pain is referred to hospital. The pain, which is relieved by the ingestion of food, is located in the upper abdomen, and a gastroenterologist concludes that there is a 30% probability that the patient has a duodenal ulcer.*

As before, we ask the clinician to substantiate his claim, and this time the clinician argues that he has studied a large number of successive patients with upper abdominal pain and that duodenoscopy revealed a duodenal ulcer in 30% of these patients.

If we imagine that the survey was so large that we need not worry about the possibility that the observed frequency differed from the true frequential probability, it is tempting to conclude that the gastroenterologist's probabilistic claim is much better substantiated than that of the cardiologist, but that is a debatable point.

In order to appreciate this problem it is necessary to remember that the gastroenterologist stated that the probability of duodenal ulcer disease in *that particular patient* was 30%. Therefore, we are concerned with a unique event, just like the maiden trip of the space-shuttle, or the result of a particular horse race. The probability was not a frequential probability, *but a subjective probability which was based on an observed frequency.* This is an important point, as the gastroenterologist need not have based his subjective belief on that particular observed frequency. He might, for instance, have taken into account that the patient in question was a woman and that the survey also showed that only 13% of women with upper abdominal pain suffered from a duodenal ulcer. Using this information, the gastroenterologist could have concluded that the probability of the diagnosis in this patient was 13%. One might also argue that even this probability is not good enough, as the gastroenterologist should have based his belief on the frequency of duodenal ulcers among female patients whose pain was relieved by food, but it is easy to see that arguments along this line invariably lead to a dead end. We might just as well ask him to base his belief on a group of patients who also had the same age, height, colour of hair and social background, and in the end the reference group would be so restricted that even the experience from a very large survey could not provide the necessary information. If we went even further and required that he must base his belief on patients who in all respects were identical with this particular patient, the probabilistic problem would vanish, as those patients, just like the patient in question, would either have or not have a duodenal ulcer. We should be dealing with a certainty rather than a probability.

The clinician's belief in a particular diagnosis in the individual patient may be based on the recorded experience in a group of patients, but it is still a subjective probability. It reflects not only the observed frequency of the disease in a reference group, but also the clinician's theoretical knowledge which determines the choice of reference group. *Recorded experience is never the sole basis of clinical decision-making.*

This discussion further illustrates the conflict between realism and empiricism, which was discussed in detail in Chapters 2 and 3. The cardiologist was a realist in so far as he based his diagnostic decision on deductions from theoretical knowledge, whereas the gastroenterologist represented the empiricist who based his decision on past experience. In practice, all clinical decisions which concern the individual patient to a varying extent contain both elements, and, considering the contemporary scientific climate, it is particularly important to note the limitation of the empiricist approach [3].

Before we leave this topic, it is worth noticing that subjective probabilities may be more or less precise. When we toss a coin our belief in the outcome 'head' is exactly 50%, but when a clinician is predicting the outcome of a particular treatment, he may simply feel that the chance of cure is somewhere around 50%. Usually this dimension of vagueness cannot be quantified but, if the clinician chooses to base his subjective belief on an observed frequency, the calculation of confidence limits may serve exactly this purpose. Imagine, for instance, that the gastroenterologist had only observed 100 patients and that thirty of those suffered from duodenal ulcer disease. In that case the statistician could have told him that the 95% confidence interval was approximately 20–40%, which means that he could be fairly certain that the true frequential probability was somewhere within that interval. Then the clinician could have stated that his personal belief in the diagnosis in that particular patient was 30±10%, and in that way he could have conveyed the information that his experience was limited, but that he felt fairly certain that even infinite experience would not affect his belief beyond those limits. The cardiologist, of course, would not be able to make a similar calculation, but he would probably think along the same lines. Those who are concerned with clinical decision theory often ask clinicians to state their subjective probability of a particular diagnosis or a particular treatment result, and it is a common experience that clinicians are unwilling to make precise estimates; they may, however, be quite happy to state that the probability of a diagnosis like myocardial infarction is, say, between 50 and 75% or between 75 and 100%.

Textbook knowledge and clinical practice

The two clinical examples which we have discussed so far were fairly straightforward. The clinician observed a patient with a particular clinical picture and assessed the subjective probability that the patient suffered from a particular disease. Such probabilities may be called *diagnostic probabilities*. Often, however, clinicians are forced to think in a roundabout way which they, themselves, are rarely able to analyse logically.

Imagine that a clinician considers the possibility that one of his patients suffers from a hepatocellular carcinoma. He requests a suitable diagnostic test, e.g. determination of α-fetoprotein in the serum, and records that it is positive. He now wishes to assess the probability of the diagnosis on the basis of this test result, but perhaps the medical literature only provides the information that a positive test is seen in 70% of patients with a hepatocellular carcinoma and in 2% of patients without this disease. How does the clinican tackle this problem? First we shall attempt a formal analysis and then we shall return to everyday clinical thinking.

The frequential probabilities which the clinician found in the

literature may in the conventional shorthand be written thus:
$P(S|D) = 0.70$ (Read: the probability of this particular sign *given* this particular disease is 70%), and
$P(S|\overline{D}) = 0.02$ (Read: the probability of this particular sign *given* the absence of this particular disease is 2%).

Such probabilities, which we shall call nosological (nosology = description and classification of diseases) are of little direct interest from a clinical point of view, as the clinician wishes to assess the 'opposite' probability. He wishes to assess $P(D|S)$, i.e. the probability of this disease *given* this sign, and the derivation of that diagnostic probability from the nosological one is not quite simple. In principle, the conversion is done by means of Bayes' theorem, which is shown below, and it is seen from the formula that in order to calculate $P(D|S)$, the clinician must know not only the nosological probabilities ($P(S|D)$ and $P(S|\overline{D})$), but also the prior probability of the presence and the absence of the disease, i.e. $P(D)$ and $P(\overline{D})$:

$$P(D|S) = \frac{P(S|D)P(D)}{P(S|D)P(D)+P(S|\overline{D})P(\overline{D})}.$$

Perhaps the clinician estimated, before he saw the positive test result, that 25% of patients with the characteristics of this particular patient suffer from hepatocellular carcinoma, i.e. $P(D) = 0.25$ and $P(\overline{D}) = 0.75$. Then he can calculate, using the formula, that the probability of the disease *given* a positive test result, $P(D|S)$, is 92%. All probabilities in this example are frequential, and $P(D|S)$ is the calculated frequency on which the clinician bases his subjective belief in the diagnosis in this particular case.

Of course, it is not suggested that clinicians make calculations of this kind, but they must in a vague sort of way think along those lines. Clinical knowledge is to a large extent based on textbook knowledge (i.e. nosology), and the ordinary textbook of medicine does not tell the reader much about the probability of different diseases given different symptoms. The textbooks are divided into chapters, one for each disease, and in these chapters the author tells the reader which symptoms and signs are very common, common or rare. In other words, the textbooks provide information of the type $P(S|D)$, and the reader cannot use this nosological information, unless in principle he uses Bayes' theorem. One may say that Bayes' theorem tells a clinician how to use textbook knowledge for practical clinical purposes.

It is not necessary for our purpose to discuss Bayes' theorem in greater detail, but it is important to note that it is impossible to convert textbook knowledge (i.e. nosological probabilities like $P(S|D)$ and $P(S|\bar{D})$) to the clinically relevant diagnostic probability, $P(D|S)$, unless the clinician is able to assess the prior probability of the presence or absence of the suspected disease. He must assess $P(D)$. The practical significance of this point is perhaps illustrated most clearly by the European doctor who accepted a position at a hospital in tropical Africa. In order to prepare himself for the new job, he bought himself a large textbook of tropical medicine and studied in great detail the clinical pictures of a large number of exotic diseases. However, for several months after his arrival at the hospital, his diagnostic performance was very poor, as he knew next to nothing about the relative frequency of all these diseases. He had to acquaint himself with the prior probability ($P(D)$) of the diseases in the catchment area of the hospital before he could make precise diagnostic assessments.

The same thing happens on a smaller scale when a doctor trained at a university hospital establishes himself in general practice. At the beginning, he will suspect his patients of all sorts of rare diseases (which are common at the university hospital), but after a while he will learn to assess correctly the frequency of different diseases in the general population.

The probability of hypotheses

Both in ordinary conversation and in science we assess not only the probability of the occurrence of particular events, but also the probability of the truth of general statements. We may say that it is *probably* true that there are living organisms in other solar systems or that it is *probably* wrong that people in the Caucasus live longer than other people. We may also quantify such statements and, for instance, say that there is a 95% probability that duodenal ulcers heal more quickly during treatment with the drug omeprazole than during treatment with another drug, cimetidine. These examples are analogous to those mentioned above when we discussed the probability of the occurrence of unique events, and once again we are dealing with *subjective* and not with frequential probabilities. The last statement does not mean, for instance, that in the long run 95% of duodenal ulcers heal during omeprazole treatment or that 95% of published trials show that omeprazole is best; it simply means that our belief in the truth of the statement is the same as our belief in picking a red marble from a bag containing ninety-five red and five white marbles; it means that we are almost, but not totally, convinced that the average healing time during omeprazole treatment is shorter than the average healing time during cimetidine treatment.

The clinician who wishes to keep abreast with the results of medical research must often make probabilistic assessments of this kind. Each week he reads a variety of medical papers and, repeatedly, he must answer questions of the following kind: Am I convinced by this evidence that lack of exercise is one of the causes of myocardial infarction? What is my confidence in the author's conclusion that ultrasonography is more reliable than CT-scanning for the diagnosis of obstructive jaundice? Do I now believe that this drug cures more patients than the drug which I use already?

The results of the majority of medical studies are quantitative, and a quarter of a century ago the clinical reader made up his mind whether or not to accept the conclusions by simply looking at the figures. If, say, twenty of twenty-five patients who received a new drug were cured, compared with twelve of twenty-five patients who received inactive tablets, the reader might conclude that this evidence strongly suggested the superiority of the new drug. He would, of course, also consider the design of the study and the results of other investigations, but in the end he might decide to introduce the new treatment on the basis of the quoted figures.

During the 1960s and '70s the presentation of scientific results gradually underwent great changes. At the beginning of that period, very few authors did a statistical analysis, but today no respectable journal will accept a paper if the results have not been subjected to statistical significance tests. The introduction of biostatistics was accompanied by a good deal of enthusiasm. A variety of elementary statistical textbooks appeared on the market, and it became fashionable to organize courses in clinical research methods in which the teaching of statistics played a dominant role. There can be little doubt that this development was long overdue and that the methodological standard of medical papers has greatly improved during the last few decades, but at the same time a new problem arose. The reading of medical journals today presupposes considerable statistical knowledge, and those doctors who are not well versed in statistical theory tend to interpret the results of significance tests uncritically or even incorrectly.

Firstly, it is often overlooked that the results of a statistical analysis depend not only on the observed data, but also on the choice of statistical model. The statistician or research worker who wishes to do a statistical analysis often has the choice between several tests which are based on different models, and it is quite possible that a t-test which assumes an underlying Gaussian distribution will show that two samples differ significantly, when a so-called rank sum test, which does not have this assumption, shows that the difference is non-significant. Unfortunately, many research workers who know little about statistics leave the statistical analysis to statisticians who know little about medicine, and the end-result may well be a series of meaningless calculations.

Secondly, many readers of medical journals do not know the correct interpretation of those P-values which are the result of significance tests. Usually, it is only stated whether the P-value is below 5% ($P < 0.05$) or above 5% ($P > 0.05$) and, according to convention, the results in the former case are said to be 'statistically significant', whereas in the latter case they are said to be 'statistically non-significant'. These expressions tend to be taken so seriously that it is almost considered 'unscientific' to believe in a 'non-significant' result or not to believe in a 'significant' result. It is sometimes taken for granted that a 'significant' difference is a true difference and that a 'non-significant' difference is a chance finding.

Of course, a distinction is also made between 'highly significant' differences ($P < 0.01$) and 'significant' ones ($0.01 < P < 0.05$), but most doctors who do concern themselves with the size of the P-values seem to interpret them in the wrong way. They tend to believe that $P < 0.05$ means that there is less than a 5% probability that there is no difference and, consequently, that there is more than a 95% probability that there is a difference. However, it should be apparent from what has been said already that this interpretation is wrong. The statement, for instance, that there is a difference between the cure rates of two treatments is a general one, and we have already pointed out that the probability of the truth of general statements—scientific hypotheses—is *subjective*, whereas the probabilities which are calculated by statisticians are frequential ones. The hypothesis that one treatment is better than the other is either true or false and cannot be interpreted in frequential terms.

In order to explain the correct interpretation of all those P-values which are found in medical journals, we shall have to introduce a little statistical theory [4].

Imagine once again that somebody found that twenty (80%) of twenty-five patients who received drug A were cured, compared with twelve (48%) of twenty-five patients who received drug B. In that case there are two possibilities: either the *null hypothesis* is true, which means that the two treatments are equally effective and the observed difference arose by chance, or the *alternative hypothesis* is true, which means that one treatment is better than the other. The clinician wants to make up his mind to what extent he believes in the truth of the alternative hypothesis (and the falsehood of the null hypothesis), and he needs the statistical analysis to help him make up his mind, but it is essential to note that the P-value does not provide a direct answer. In this case the statistician would probably do a so-called Fisher's test which would give the result that $P = 4\%$, meaning that the difference is 'statistically significant' ($P < 0.05$), but, as explained already, that does not mean that there is a 4% probability that the null hypothesis is true (and that there is a 96% probability that the alternative hypothesis is true). The P-value is a frequential probability and it provides the information that there is a 4% probability of obtaining such a difference between the cure rates, *if* the null hypothesis is true. In other words, the statistician asks us to assume that the null hypothesis is true and to imagine that we do a large number of trials. In that case, the long-run frequency of trials which show a difference between the cure rates like the one we found, or an even larger one (i.e. a difference of 32% or more), will be 4%.

In order to explain the implications of the correct statistical definition of a P-value, we shall first imagine that the patients who took part in this particular trial suffered from a duodenal ulcer, and that drug A was ascorbic acid, while drug B was a placebo preparation (inactive tablets). If that was the case, we should reason somewhat along these lines: our theoretical knowledge gives us no grounds for believing that ascorbic acid has any effect whatsoever on the healing of duodenal ulcers, for which reason our prior confidence in the null hypothesis is immense, whereas our prior confidence in the alternative hypothesis is minute. Perhaps our degree of belief in the null hypothesis is 99.99%, i.e. the same as our belief in picking a red marble from a bag containing 9999 red ones and one white one, whereas our belief in the alternative hypothesis is 0.01% (i.e. the same as our belief in picking the white marble from that bag).

We must take these prior probabilities into account when we assess the result of the trial, and we have the following choice: either we accept the null hypothesis, in spite of the fact that the probability of the trial result is fairly low (4%) if the null hypothesis is true, or we accept the alternative hypothesis in spite of the fact that the probability of that hypothesis is judged to be extremely low (about 0.01%) in the light of our prior knowledge.

It is seen that the choice is a difficult one, as both hypotheses, each in its own way, may be said to be unlikely, but we believe that any clinician who reasons along these lines will choose that hypothesis which is least unacceptable: he will accept the null hypothesis and suggest that the difference between the cure rates arose by chance, as he does not feel that the evidence from this single trial is sufficient to shake his prior belief in the null hypothesis.

Compare this balanced argument with that of the clinician who erroneously believes that the P-value is simply the probability of the truth of the null hypothesis. He will conclude that this single trial provides the information that it is 96% certain that ascorbic acid promotes ulcer healing [5].

Alternatively, we may imagine that the quoted figures originated from a duodenal ulcer trial, in which drug A was a new H_2-receptor blocker (which inhibits the acid secretion in the stomach) and drug B, as before, a placebo preparation. In that case our prior belief in the null hypothesis and the alternative hypothesis would be very different. We know that other H_2-blockers greatly enhance ulcer healing, and, if laboratory experiments have shown that the new drug inhibits acid secretion just as effectively as the old ones, we shall have great confidence in the alternative hypothesis and little confidence in the null hypothesis. Therefore, the final verdict in this case presents few problems, as both our prior knowledge and the results of the statistical analysis point against the null hypothesis, and we shall certainly end up by concluding that there is very little doubt that the drug is effective. If we were asked to quantify our subjective belief in the alternative hypothesis, we might say that we feel more than 99% sure that it is true. In contrast, the doctor who erroneously interprets the P-value as the probability of the truth of the null hypothesis, would also have to conclude in this case that it is 96% certain that the drug is effective.

It will be noticed that these arguments have much in common with diagnostic reasoning, using Bayes' theorem. The P-value is the frequential probability of the observed data *given* the truth of the null hypothesis, and the doctor who wishes to draw the correct conclusion from the scientific investigation tries to assess the (subjective) probability that the null hypothesis is true *given* the observed data. In much the same way as the diagnostician, he is concerned with the conversion of a conditional probability, which requires that he takes into account the prior probability. Some statistical decision theorists, who believe that Bayes' theorem is also valid for the computation of subjective probabilities, have asserted that it is possible to calculate the probability of the truth of a hypothesis [6, 7], but these methods which are controversial will not be discussed here.

These reflections on the interpretation of statistical tests and the importance of prior beliefs also have philosophical implications, as they reveal that empirical natural science is never theory-free, and probably never value-free. We may do our very best to ensure that our investigations are not biased by our beliefs, hopes and expectations, but the quantitative results which we publish must ultimately be interpreted in the light of our prior beliefs. The probability of the truth or falsehood of a scientific hypothesis is subjective, which means that we cannot eliminate the subjective factor when we decide which hypothesis was confirmed and which was refuted.

The conclusions also agree well with one of Kuhn's theses. Kuhn has pointed out that scientists tend to ignore results which are at variance with those theories which are part of the paradigm of a science. They only abandon a theory when a considerable amount of contradictory evidence has accumulated (see p. 5). In this

Probability and Belief 103

chapter we have presented the same idea, using different words. Scientists who interpret the results of statistical tests correctly will not accept the first study which produces unexpected results, as their prior belief in the suggested conclusion is small. If, however, successive studies give similar results, their prior belief in the hypothesis will increase gradually, and in the end the scientific community will be convinced.

Notes and references

1 The exact confidence limits which are quoted in these examples are derived from the binomial distribution. Tables of confidence limits are included in, for example, Diem, K. & Lentner, C. (eds) *Scientific Tables Geigy,* 7th edn. Basle: Geigy, 1970.
2 The presentation of the probability concept in this chapter is much simplified. As mentioned below, Bayesian statistical theory also takes into account subjective probabilities [6, 7]. Probability theory, which is closely linked to the problem of induction (Chapter 2), has attracted the interest of a number of empiricist philosophers, e.g. Rudolf Carnap (1891–1970) and R. E. von Mises (1883–1953), but it is beyond the scope of this book to discuss the topic in greater depth. For our purpose it is sufficient to distinguish between frequential and subjective probabilities.
3 Computer diagnosis is the best example of the extreme empiricist approach to diagnostic problems. The computer is fed with information about the clinical pictures of a large number of patients and, on the basis of this experience, it is possible to calculate the probability of different diagnoses in future cases, for instance by means of Bayesian logic (see Note 7). In some restricted areas this method has proved very successful (see, for instance, de Dombal, F.T. Surgical diagnosis assisted by a computer. *Proceedings of the Royal Society London (B),* 1973; **84**: 433–40). It is, however, typical of such studies that they are confined to diagnoses which can be verified, for instance, by surgical operation. For reasons already explained, no computer can calculate the probability of a disease like myocardial infarction on the basis of recorded experience.
4 Here we shall discuss the interpretation of significance tests, but as mentioned on p. 44, it is also possible to calculate the confidence limits of the difference between two cure rates (see Wulff, H.R. Confidence limits in evaluating controlled therapeutic trials. *Lancet,* 1973; **11**: 969–70).
5 Misinterpretation of *P*-values is extremely common. At an advanced course in research methods in Denmark, twenty-five doctors were asked what is meant by a *P*-value, and all of them believed that it was the probability of the truth of the null hypothesis. One of the reasons for this state of affairs may well be that those who teach research methods do not themselves appreciate the problem. For instance, S. A. Glanz writes in his paper 'Biostatistics: how to detect, correct and prevent errors in the medical literature' (*Circulation,* 1980; **61**: 1–6): 'Precisely, the *P*-value is the probability of obtaining a value of the test statistic as large or larger than the one computed from the data when in reality there is no difference

between the different treatments. In other words the *P*-value is the probability of being wrong when asserting that a difference exists.' The first statement in this quotation is a correct interpretation of the frequential meaning of a *P*-value, whereas the second statement is a *non sequitur*.

6 Lindley, D. *Making Decisions*. London: Wiley Interscience, 1973.
7 Winkler, R.L. *Introduction to Bayesian Inference and Decision*. New York: Holt, Rinehart and Winston, 1972.

CHAPTER 8
THE NATURALISTIC APPROACH TO PSYCHIATRY

Contemporary medicine in general has its critics who doubt the ability of the medical profession to cope with the health problems of modern society, but psychiatry is the only medical discipline which enjoys the doubtful honour of facing a veritable protest movement. Some members of this movement, e.g. Laing, Szasz and Foudraine, have little in common philosophically, but they are united in their radical criticism of psychiatry, both as a science and as a social institution, and their stance, which is known as *anti-psychiatry* [1], has from time to time received much attention in the news media. It is claimed by these critics that mental diseases are not diseases in the ordinary medical sense, and Szasz, for instance, writes:

> It is customary to define psychiatry as a medical speciality concerned with the study, diagnosis and treatment of mental illnesses. This is a worthless and misleading definition. Mental illness is a myth. Psychiatrists are not concerned with mental illnesses and their treatment. In actual practice they deal with personal, social and ethical problems in living [2].

The anti-psychiatrists also remind us that it is tempting to exclude dissidents from the community, if their opinions and behaviour constitute a threat to the order of society, and they claim that psychiatry has proved an excellent tool for the suppression of such people; first, the dissidents are declared ill and, next, they are rendered innocuous by drug treatment and electroconvulsive therapy. Laing has expressed this point of view as follows:

> There is no such 'condition' as 'schizophrenia', but the label is

a social fact and the social fact is a *political event*.... The
person labeled is inaugurated not only into a role, but into a
career of patient, by the concerted action of a coalition (a
'conspiracy') of family, of GP, mental health officer,
psychiatrists, nurses, psychiatric social workers, and often
fellow patients. The 'committed' person labeled as patient,
and specifically as 'schizophrenic', is degraded from full
existential and legal status as human agent and responsible
person to someone no longer in possession of his own
definition of himself, unable to retain his own possessions,
precluded from the exercise of his discretion as to whom he
meets, what he does. His time is no longer his own, and the
space he occupies is no longer of his choosing [3].

The anti-psychiatric movement has found many of its followers among psychologists, sociologists and writers, whereas most psychiatrists have felt that the criticism is too radical and too crude. Van Praag, for instance, has retaliated in the following way:

Anti-psychiatrists created a certain climate in psychiatry:
romantic, anti-intellectual, dogmatic and anti-
methodological—complete with hero-worship (Laing,
Cooper, Szasz, Foudraine and others). Feeling, intuition,
empathy, encounter, sensitivity, spontaneity were praised as
superior to such concepts as analysis, verification and
evaluation [4].

The debate, however, has had the beneficial effect that psychiatrists in their attempt to counter the attacks have been forced to reflect on the philosophical basis of their own discipline. They have had to consider the *epistemological* question: How does one recognize mental disease? and they have had to ask the *ontological* question: What is the true nature of mental disease? Is it, for example, a biochemical disturbance, or is it, as some anti-psychiatrists claim, an expression of a social conflict? However, as usual, it is difficult in practice to distinguish sharply between these two levels of philosophical discourse.

How does one recognize mental disease?

In Chapter 4 we discussed the mechanical model of disease, and it was mentioned that, according to Boorse, disease is regarded as a deviation from the *species design*. A person is said to be ill when the functions of his body are found to be depressed below species-typical levels. The Danish philosopher of law, Alf Ross, who was particularly concerned with the epistemological aspects of the disease concept, arrived at the same conclusion as Boorse regarding somatic disease, and he also endeavoured to define mental disease in much the same manner [5]. Just as we presuppose a species-typical level with regard to biological function, Ross presupposes a species-typical level with regard to the ability of man to communicate with others, and he regards a person as mentally ill when this ability is depressed below the species-typical level. In other words, mental disease is a condition which interferes with communication, and Ross distinguishes between two important kinds of communication disturbances: *cognitive* disturbances, like hallucinations and delusions, and *emotional–conative* disturbances (conative = related to voluntary action), like anxiety, depression and impulsiveness. Persons who exhibit such disturbances are mentally ill, as the impairment of their ability to communicate will lead to isolation and alienation; in severe cases they may even perish, if they do not receive the necessary help. According to Ross, a person who claims that the mafia governs his actions by means of rays directed at his brain, is objectively ill, as the delusions will prevent normal contact with other people.

However, many psychiatrists will disagree with Ross when he claims that he has established an objective criterion for the distinction between mental disease and mental health. It is true, of course, that the ability to communicate is important and that many psychiatric patients are deeply worried about their isolation, but it is a matter of doubt whether Ross's criterion of mental illness can be used in practice. It seems highly unlikely that it will ever be possible to obtain sufficient consensus among psychiatrists regarding the presence or absence of a species-typical ability to communicate in the individual case, and it may even be argued that the very idea of a species-typical ability to communicate with others is an illusion. It was concluded in Chapter 4 that normality of biological functions in the last resort depends on personal and cultural norms, and normal behaviour differs so much in different cultural settings that the same conclusion seems almost inevitable in the case of the normality of communication among people.

Therefore, it is only natural that some psychiatrists are *conventionalists,* i.e. they claim that the distinction between mental disease and mental health is dictated by those conventions which characterize a particular culture. Otherwise it is difficult to explain that homosexuality [6], which is now looked upon as a sexual variant, was once regarded as a mental disease, and that political dissidents in some parts of the world are diagnosed as suffering from paranoia in need of psychiatric treatment.

Others who, like Ross, object to the idea that psychiatric practice, to a greater extent than other branches of medicine, reflects current fashion, cultural tradition and political power, assert that in principle there is no difference between the diagnosis of mental illness and somatic illness. Emil Kraepelin (1856–1926), for instance, who is one of the founders of modern psychiatry, claimed that mental diseases are characterized by a specific cause, a particular cerebral pathology, a particular clinical picture and a specific treatment. However, as explained previously (Chapters 5 and 6) this simplistic view is not even tenable in somatic medicine.

We shall now present four current views of mental disease, including the empiricist view which reflects most clearly the conventionalist attitude, and the biological view which underlines the close relationship between psychiatry and somatic medicine. The empiricists, as might be expected, refrain from ontological considerations, whereas the other traditions reflect different views of the nature of mental illness.

The empiricist view

The followers of the critical clinical school, which is closely associated with the empiricist tradition (Chapter 3), claim that it is necessary to test the efficacy of different treatments of different diseases by means of randomized controlled trials, and they point out that the application of the results of such trials requires that doctors everywhere diagnose their patients according to the same rules. They do not concern themselves with metaphysical questions, such as the true meaning of words like health and disease, and accept the conventional disease classification without much discussion, but they stress the importance of precise definitions of individual disease entities.

This mode of thought has been accepted by many psychiatrists [7], and the much used *Diagnostic and Statistical Manual of Mental Disorders,* published by the American Psychiatric Association, is a good example [8]. The authors have defined a large number of mental disorders from an operational point of view, making as few assumptions as possible regarding the aetiology, the pathogenesis and the psychological interpretation of the symptoms. They base their definitions on those symptoms and signs which the patients present, and their aim is to facilitate those empirical investigations which are needed to increase our factual knowledge and to treat our patients more effectively.

Let us consider more closely a single example from the manual: *Generalized anxiety disorder,* which is regarded as one of several *anxiety disorders,* is diagnosed when a patient presents symptoms from at least three of the following four categories of symptoms:

1 Motor tension (i.e. shakiness, trembling, muscle aches, fatigability, etc.).
2 Autonomic hyperactivity (i.e. sweating, heart pounding, dizziness, diarrhoea, flushing, etc.).
3 Apprehensive expectation (i.e. anxiety, worry, fear, rumination, etc.).
4 Vigilance and scanning (i.e. hyperattentiveness, insomnia, irritability, impotence, etc.).

In addition, it is required that the patient must have had the symptoms for more than one month, that the patient is at least eighteen years old, and that he or she does not have symptoms which are attributed to other diseases, e.g. schizophrenia.

This is a typical example of an attempt to establish a theory-free, purely descriptive definition of a disease entity in psychiatry, and those who do randomized controlled trials may use such definitions to select their patients. We shall not discuss here whether this particular definition is sufficiently precise to warrant that use.

Psychiatrists, wishing to refine empirical studies of mental illness, have also attempted to *quantify* the severity of psychiatric symptoms. The British psychiatrist Max Hamilton, for instance, has constructed a rating-scale for measuring anxiety [9]. The scale takes into account fourteen items, including anxious mood, tension, fears and autonomic symptoms. The severity of each of these is recorded on a five-point scale and the total anxiety score is the sum of the scores for each item. Hamilton has also constructed a rating-scale for the measurement of depression [10], which is often used in controlled trials for assessing the effect of antidepressive drugs. New rating-scales must be thoroughly tested before they are introduced into clinical practice, and it is necessary to consider both the inter-observer agreement when different psychiatrists examine the same patient and the validity of the scale, i.e. the extent to which the scale measures what it is supposed to measure. The latter question can, of course, rarely be answered in exact terms.

The empiricist approach has helped to clarify one of the issues of the anti-psychiatry debate. It follows from the anti-psychiatrists' view of schizophrenia that it is considered possible, by means of intensive psychotherapy, to draw schizophrenic patients out of their psychotic state and at the same time induce personal maturation and increased creativity [11]. That claim is regarded as provocative by most British and Scandinavian psychiatrists who, according to the tradition which stems from Kraepelin, regard schizophrenia as a disease which cannot be cured, although some of the symptoms may be alleviated, for instance by drug treatment. However, this debate, which took place on both sides of the Atlantic, lost its impetus when it was recognized that the diagnostic term, schizophrenia, is used differently in different parts of the world. R. E. Kendell [12] reports a study which includes 175 admissions to mental hospitals supplying Greater London, and 192 to state hospitals supplying New York City. Sixty-two per cent of the American patients were said to suffer from schizophrenia, whereas this was only the case in 34% of the British patients, but, when the diagnostic criteria were standardized, the difference disappeared completely. Other studies also confirm that in Europe many of those patients, who in the United States are said to be schizophrenic, are diagnosed as neurosis, depression, mania or personality disorder [13]. It is well accepted in Europe that neurotic patients may respond to intensive psychotherapy, and it is obviously absurd to continue the 'anti-psychiatry' debate and to discuss the relative importance of social and genetic factors until it has been made quite clear which patients the debaters are talking about.

The definition of disease entities for the purpose of controlled therapeutic research is an important matter, but the empiricist belief that it is possible to solve all the problems of psychiatric practice by means of theory-free empirical research is unwarranted. It is necessary to test new treatments critically, but the choice between drug treatment, behaviour therapy and psychoanalysis in a case of 'generalized anxiety disorder' is not only a question of the relative efficiency of these treatments; the choice also reflects the psychiatrist's view of the nature of mental illness. Everybody practising psychiatry, even those who regard themselves as empiricists, make ontological assumptions, and we believe that these assumptions must be analysed and discussed openly so that they are not left to the personal intuition of the individual doctor. We shall now present three different theories concerning the true nature of mental disease.

Mental disease as abnormal biological function

Psychiatry is regarded as a medical discipline and, in order to justify this fact, it is sometimes claimed that mental diseases, just like somatic diseases, can be described and analysed in accordance with the biological disease concept, i.e. the mechanical model. Of course, the symptoms of mental disease differ from those of somatic diseases, but it is assumed that mental or behavioural disturbances are determined by physiological or biochemical abnormalities in the central nervous system. This point of view presupposes a definition of normal species-typical function of the central nervous system and, therefore, the advocates of biological psychiatry face the same philosophical problems as those colleagues who practise internal medicine or surgery (Chapter 4).

The dependency of mental phenomena on brain structure and function is so well known that a detailed discussion is unwarranted. It is, for instance, well established that brain lesions may cause mental disease and behavioural changes, and that biochemical dysfunction may be associated with mental symptoms. A drug like LSD may cause an acute psychotic syndrome, and withdrawal of barbiturates from chronically intoxicated persons may provoke classical psychotic symptoms, including disorientation, hallucinations and delusions.

The popularity of biological psychiatry reached its peak in the 1950s, when chlorpromazine was introduced for the treatment of psychoses. Psychiatric patients were discharged wholesale from mental hospitals and it was felt by many that the scientific revolution had at long last reached psychiatry, but, later, psychiatrists became more aware of the side-effects of treatment, and it now looks as if the improved treatment results in the 1950s were due not only to the new pharmacotherapy, but also to the activation of the patients. Nevertheless, there can be little doubt that the course of many psychiatric disorders is influenced by drug treatment. In manic-depressive psychosis, for instance, tricyclic compounds and monoamine oxidase inhibitors have an antidepressant effect, lithium has a prophylactic effect, and reserpine may provoke depression.

The biological model is not only supported by empirical clinical studies, but also by new theoretical, neurobiological knowledge about synaptic transmission and drug action on the molecular level. It has been shown, for instance, that benzodiazepines react with specific receptors in the central nervous system and, probably, these receptors play an important role when the benzodiazepines exert their anxiolytic effect [14, 15]. It also seems likely that the 'benzodiazepine receptors' play a physiological role in brain function by mediating the effect of endogenous chemical substances [16], and on this background it is possible to discern the outlines of a biological theory concerning states of anxiety. Perhaps genetically determined differences in the structure of the 'benzodiazepine receptors' have the effect that some people are less resistant to psycho-social stress and more prone to developing a state of anxiety than others [17].

In spite of such conjectures, it remains a fact that at present the biological disease concept is better founded in psychotic conditions than in neuroses and personality disorders. Most psychiatrists agree that psychoses are diseases in a medical sense and that psychotic patients must be treated by medical doctors, but some admit that possibly neuroses and personality disorders are treated more adequately by psychologists.

Mental disease as inappropriate behaviour

Presently, we shall consider a totally different approach to the problems of clinical psychiatry, but first it is necessary to write a little about the background. As we shall discuss in greater detail in the last chapter of this book, the British philosopher Gilbert Ryle (1900–76) made the radical claim that all statements about mental phenomena can be analysed in terms of statements about dispositions to different kinds of behaviour. The feeling of hunger is no more than 'hunger behaviour' and the feeling of anxiety is 'anxiety behaviour'. That philosophical theory, which is called *logical behaviourism,* appeals to the empiricist scientist, as it reduces subjective feelings to observable events, and it is mentioned here as it may be regarded as the philosophical counterpart of *behaviourism in psychology,* which is associated with such names as Ivan Pavlov, J. B. Watson and B. F. Skinner.

At the turn of the century, Pavlov (1849–1936) demonstrated the importance of the process which is now called *classical conditioning.* Dogs usually respond to the sight or smell of food by increased salivation, and, in his well-known experiments, Pavlov conditioned dogs to respond in the same manner to the sounding of a bell; he established *a conditioned reflex* by associating the offering of food with the sound of the bell. Skinner (b. 1904) also studied the behaviour of animals under experimental conditions, but extended his ideas to the analysis of human behaviour. He took a particular interest in the 'teaching' of new forms of behaviour by manipulating the consequences, and he believes that those mechanisms which he observed in the laboratory also play a major role in the natural development of the complex behaviour patterns of human beings. A particular kind of behaviour can, for instance, be strengthened if it is associated with a reward *(positive reinforcement),* it can be weakened or abolished (extinguished) if it is not positively reinforced or if it is associated with something unpleasant *(negative reinforcement)* [18]. Skinner completely rejects the idea that mental states can *cause* behaviour, e.g. that it is the feeling of hunger which induces a person to eat. It is the lack of food which induces a particular physiological state, and it is that state which, as the result of a conditioning process, makes the person go to the kitchen and take some food. The feeling of hunger is just a collateral product of the physiological state.

However, it must be emphasized that few contemporary psychologists endorse Skinner's radical views, and new versions of behaviourism are being developed which acknowledge the importance of the inner states of the central nervous system and cognitive processes.

These are the philosophical and psychological theories which form the background of modern *behaviourist psychiatry*. It is, of course, difficult to imagine a psychiatrist who would agree with Skinner that the mental life of human beings can be ignored—for which reason behaviourism in psychiatry is more closely related to modern behaviourist theories than to the classical ones—but ardent behaviourists among psychiatrists do claim that, in principle, there is no difference between a neurosis and other forms of acquired behaviour. Both appropriate and inappropriate patterns of behaviour are the result of a learning process, and the treatment of inappropriate behaviour, *behaviour therapy*, must be based on modern theories of learning.

'Neurotic anxiety', for instance, is regarded as a complex kind of behaviour which has subjective, autonomic and skeletal motor components (e.g. the feeling of anxiety, sweating and trembling), and it is assumed that this behaviour has been established by the process of classical conditioning. People usually show anxiety behaviour when they are threatened, but in the neurotic patient the conditioning has had the effect that anxiety is also evoked by stimuli which in others do not have this effect ('stimulus generalization'). Furthermore, the conditioned anxiety has the property of an acquired drive which elicits and reinforces avoidance behaviour, as the escape response to anxiety-provoking stimuli is followed by anxiety reduction. In these ways 'anxiety behaviour' of the neurotic patient in his daily life is as inappropriate as the 'hunger behaviour' of a Pavlovian dog which reacts to the sound of a bell.

Behaviour therapy has gained ground in psychiatry in recent years, particularly for the treatment of non-psychotic conditions like neuroses, sexual problems, alcoholism and drug addiction. A person with anxiety neurosis may, for instance, be treated by *systematic desensitization,* which means that the person is exposed to a series of carefully graded anxiety-provoking situations; in this way the conditioned anxiety is extinguished, and the patient 'cured'. Other therapeutic principles may also be used, such as *aversion therapy* (i.e. extinction of undesirable behaviour by associating the stimulus which elicits the behaviour with an aversive one), *token economy* (i.e. positive reinforcement of desirable behaviour by token rewards), *social skills training,* and *progressive muscular relaxation* [19]. Some of these treatments seem to be effective when they are tested by means of the principles of the critical clinical school.

Behaviour therapy is used by convinced behaviourists who assert that it only serves to mystify the issue when conditions, like a neurosis or alcoholism, are regarded as diseases in the medical sense, but, of course, the same therapeutic principles can also be used by psychiatrists who trust their efficiency, but reject the implications of the underlying theory.

Mental disease as a social problem

The 'anti-psychiatrists' go much too far when they characterize mental disease as a healthy response to a sick society, but there is a nucleus of truth in their criticism of biological psychiatry, as there can be no doubt that social factors play an important role in the development of mental—as well as somatic—disease. Some psychiatrists who also stress this point study scientifically the influence of the social environment and regard at least some mental conditions as social problems. A drug addict, for instance, may present certain psychological and biological characteristics, but from the point of view of *social psychiatry,* the essential features of drug addiction are those factors in society which determine the development and dissemination of the 'disease'. H. S. Becker [20], for instance, has pointed out that the use of marijuana in Western societies is associated with participation in certain subcultures. Those who are accepted as members of such subcultures have gone through a process of socialization during which they have learned to accept certain rules, norms and customs, and the use of marijuana is part of that pattern of life. From this point of view, the study of the marijuana habit is tantamount to the study of those factors which determined the emergence of those subcultures in industrial societies after the Second World War, and, therefore, social psychiatry is closely related to social medicine and to sociology (Chapter 10).

The biological, psychological (behaviouristic) and social traditions reflect different ontological views—different views of the nature of mental disease—and the choice between them has practical implications. The followers of the first two traditions will advocate treatment of the individual patient by means of behaviour therapy or drugs, whereas social psychiatrists will favour preventive measures directed against groups of individuals, and it may be argued that intervention at that level is a socio-political rather than a medical problem.

The choice of disease concept also determines the status of psychiatry. If we accept the biological model, there is no doubt whatsoever that psychiatry is a medical discipline, but, if we accept one of the other models, psychiatry might as well be regarded as a branch of psychology or sociology.

The eclectic view

In this chapter we have tried to give a systematic account of a number of views of modern psychiatry, but probably we have gone too far in our attempts to simplify and systematize the presentation.

We have used the points of view of the anti-psychiatrists to exemplify the contemporary criticism of psychiatric practice, but the current debate about the status of psychiatry is much more varied. It is true that some critics, like the anti-psychiatrists, claim that the biological concept of mental disease is a dangerous illusion, as it leads to drug treatment of existential problems and serves to gloss over the social inequalities and cultural problems of industrialized societies. But it must also be remembered that many people demand that their doctor writes a prescription when they suffer nervous symptoms, and that other critics claim that psychiatric patients are discriminated against because mental diseases are not accorded the same status as somatic diseases.

We have described four different schools of thought within the community of psychiatrists and we may have left the impression that the distinctions between these views are sharper than they really are. But we shall maintain that the paradigm of psychiatry is much less established than that of most other branches of medicine, and it appears that the differences of opinion among psychiatrists reflect three philosophical problems.

The first of these concerns the distinction between mental disease and mental health. As discussed above, those psychiatrists who are influenced by empiricist thinking do not concern themselves with the nature of mental disease, but adopt the conventionalist attitude that mental disease is what psychiatrists treat, whereas biologically orientated psychiatrists, who believe that mental disease is a deviation from species-typical normality, contend that it is a question of objective truth whether or not a particular patient is mentally ill.

The second philosophical problem concerns the theoretical frame of reference. We have distinguished between the biological, psychological (behaviouristic) and social concepts of mental disease, and we have mentioned the practical implications of the issue. Many psychiatrists, however, will feel that this distinction is artificial and that the three 'disease concepts' are just three aspects of one holistic concept of mental illness. It has often been claimed in recent years that it is necessary to use a holistic *bio-psycho-social model* of mental disease, as one must pay equal respect to biological, psychological and social factors in order to attain a comprehensive characterization of the individual patient. It is impossible in clinical practice to confine oneself to, for instance, the biological concept, as psychiatric patients, just like other persons, are unique human beings in terms of biological function, psychological characteristics and social background. A psychiatrist may decide to sedate an anxious patient with delirium tremens, but that does not imply a disregard of those psycho-social factors which determined that the patient became an alcoholic. Pariser *et al.*, in a discussion of the causes of anxiety, express the holistic view in the following way:

> We will emphasize that the experience of anxiety is a multi-determined event resulting from the development of genetic potential, most likely mediated by individual variations of cellular neurotransmitter systems under the influence of multiple psychosocial factors [21].

However, it also remains a fact that some psychiatrists have committed themselves to one particular school of thought and, therefore, contemporary psychiatry is characterized by both *reductionist* and *eclectic* [22] tendencies. The reductionists, i.e. those who reduce mental illness to biological abnormalities, behavioural disturbances or social problems, only take into account one aspect of the disease mechanism, but, by doing so, they secure themselves a theoretical frame of reference which permits them to formulate fruitful theories and to carry out scientific investigations, which may lead to improved treatment of psychiatric patients [23].

The *eclectics* who adopt the bio-psycho-social model, the elements of which have been drawn from three theoretical systems, may do well in clinical practice, but their approach is unsatisfactory from both a philosophical and a scientific point of view. As pointed out by Kuhn, a scientific concept only acquires meaning in the context of the paradigm to which it belongs, and a disease model which borrows concepts from three different paradigms is an unsatisfactory starting point for the formulation of fruitful theories.

The third philosophical controversy has yet to be discussed: Is psychiatry a natural science or does it belong to the human sciences? The followers of all the schools of thought which we have discussed so far, including both reductionists and eclectics, take it for granted that mental diseases, just like other natural phenomena, can be observed, described and classified by means of empirical methods. They also agree that, in principle, mental illness can be explained by demonstrating its causes, even though they disagree about the true nature of those causes. Therefore, all the models of mental disease which have been discussed in this chapter represent variants of *naturalistic psychiatry*, i.e. psychiatry as a natural science. In the following chapters we shall consider the alternative point of view that the naturalistic concept of man is grossly inadequate and that the study of mental and social phenomena requires a radically different approach.

Notes and references

1 The anti-psychiatry movement has no well-defined programme, except that most anti-psychiatrists reject the medical disease model. Their position is well presented in the critical reviews by H. M. van Praag [4] and M. S. Moore (Some myths about 'mental illness'. *Archives of General Psychiatry*, 1975; 32: 1483–97).
2 Szasz, T.S. *The Myth of Mental Illness*. New York: Del Publishing Co., 1961, p. 296.
3 Laing, R.D. *The Politics of Experience*. New York: Pantheon, 1967, pp. 83–4.
4 Praag, H.M. van. The scientific foundation of anti-psychiatry. *Acta Psychiatrica Scandinavica*, 1978; 58: 113–41.

5 Ross, A. Det psykopatologiske sygdomsbegreb. (The psychopathological concept of disease. In Danish.) *Bibliotek for Læger*, 1980; **172**: 1–23.
6 We are referring to ego-syntonic homosexuality, i.e. homosexuality which is accepted by the individuals in question. Ego-dystonic homosexuality, i.e. homosexuality which constitutes a permanent source of distress to the persons in question, is still regarded as a mental disorder in the *Diagnostic and Statistical Manual of Mental Disorders* [8].
7 *Archives of General Psychiatry* and *British Journal of Psychiatry* contain numerous examples of empiricist research.
8 *Diagnostic and Statistical Manual of Mental Disorders*, 3rd edn. Washington: American Psychiatric Association, 1980.
9 Hamilton, M. The assessment of anxiety states by rating. *British Journal of Medical Psychology*, 1959; **32**: 50–5.
10 Hamilton, M. A rating scale for depression. *Journal of Neurology, Neurosurgery and Psychiatry*, 1960; **23**: 56–62.
11 See, for instance, the story of Mary Barnes. She is the most eloquent witness of the Laingian movement, supporting their use of psychotherapeutic techniques (Barnes, M. & Berke, J. *Mary Barnes: Two Accounts of a Journey Through Madness*). Harmondsworth: Penguin Books, 1973.
12 Kendell, R.E. *The Role of Diagnosis in Psychiatry*. Oxford: Blackwell Scientific Publications, 1975, p. 72.
13 pp. 74–7 in [12].
14 Squires, R.F. & Braestrup, C. Benzodiazepine receptors in rat brain. *Nature*, 1977; **266**: 732–4.
15 Möhler, H. & Okada, T. Benzodiazepine receptors: demonstration in the central nervous system. *Science*, 1977; **198**: 849–51.
16 Insel, T.R., Ninan, P.T., Aloi, J., Jimerson, D.C., Skolnick, P. & Paul, S.M. A benzodiazepine receptor-mediated model of anxiety. *Archives of General Psychiatry*, 1984; **41**: 741–50.
17 Until recently 'panic disorder' [8] was interpreted almost exclusively in psychological terms. It was believed that the patients were overreacting to life stress or to an unconscious conflict. An alternative theory has been suggested, according to which panic disorder is associated with a biochemical abnormality in the central nervous system (Sheehan, D.V. Panic attacks and phobias. *New England Journal of Medicine*, 1982; **307**: 156–8).
18 It should be noticed that there is some terminological confusion in the literature. According to Skinner, for instance, negative reinforcement is not weakening of a certain behaviour by punishment, but strengthening of a certain behaviour by removal of an unpleasant stimulus. (See, for instance: Skinner, B.F. *About Behaviourism*. London: Jonathan Cape, 1974, p. 46.) Strengthening of avoidance behaviour by anxiety reduction is a good example of negative reinforcement in Skinner's terminology.
19 Meyer, V. & Chesser, E.S. *Behavior Therapy in Clinical Psychiatry*. Harmondsworth: Penguin Books, 1970, p. 50.
20 Becker, H.S. *Outsiders*. New York: The Free Press of Glencoe, 1963.
21 Pariser, S.F., Pinta, E.R., Jones, B.A. & Young, E.A. Diagnosis and management of anxiety symptoms and syndromes. In: Davis, J.M. & Greenblatt, D. (eds) *Psychopharmacology, Update; New and Neglected Areas*. New York: Grune & Stratton, 1979, p. 145.

22 An eclectic is somebody who selects and combines principles and opinions belonging to different schools of thought. Therefore, the bio-psycho-social model is an eclectic theory.
23 It may be noted as a matter of curiosity that the anti-psychiatrists are extreme reductionists when they assert, as Laing does, that mental illness is no more than a reflection of social conflicts and conspiracies.

CHAPTER 9
HERMENEUTICS: THE NATURE OF MAN IN A WIDER PERSPECTIVE

*I*n the preceding chapters medicine has been regarded almost exclusively as a branch of natural science, and the philosophical discussion has largely been confined to the two traditions in the philosophy of science which were labelled empiricism and realism.

In this chapter we wish to introduce the reader to some of the ideas of a very different philosophical tradition, and we shall defend the point of view that the naturalistic concept of man is unacceptably simplistic and narrow as it ignores some of the most important constituent features of human nature. We shall not deny, of course, that man is a biological organism, but we shall argue that man is *more than* a biological organism and that medicine is *more than* a branch of natural science. This is a very complex philosophical issue and in order not to get lost in sophisticated philosophical arguments, we shall concentrate on one particular topic, *the concept of anxiety,* which is of paramount importance from both a medical and a philosophical point of view.

This is a familiar topic, in so far as everybody knows what it means to be afraid. It is easy for most people to recall situations when their body was in a tumult: the heart was throbbing and the hands were cold and moist; it was felt that the situation was getting out of control and the mental condition was one of alarm. In most such instances it presents no problem at all to identify the cause of the emotional reaction, for instance in the form of impending physical danger, and under such circumstances fear may be regarded as a normal constituent of our elementary defence mechanisms. This is what may be called *rational fear*.

There are also some people who suffer from irrational fear, which means that they experience this emotion under specific circumstances which are not usually considered threatening. Such irrational fear is called a *phobia*, and claustrophobia is the classical example. Phobias are of particular interest to psychoanalysts, and we shall return to that topic in Chapter 11.

Here, however, we shall not concern ourselves with rational fear and phobias, but with a third kind of fear which has no identifiable cause. We are referring to those people who suffer from a persistent feeling of unexplained *anxiety*, which in some cases may reach such degrees that the person's ability to function socially is seriously compromised. Anxiety of this kind is a common problem in psychiatric practice as illustrated by the fact that it constitutes a recognized mental disorder (p. 109), but it is equally interesting in this context that such anxiety is also an important philosophical concept. A number of philosophers, especially on the continent of Europe, have concerned themselves with the mood which in philosophical literature is often called *angst*, and this word means much the same as unexplained anxiety in the language of psychiatrists [1].

We shall approach the topic by means of a clinical example. A middle-aged woman seeks specialist advice because of nervous symptoms. She is a divorced housewife and can no longer see the purpose of her life. Her children, who are grown-up, have left the home, and she has also lost her friends as she dares not go out on her own. Therefore, she is alone much of the time, and she finds herself in a state of persistent anxiety. The psychiatrist who sees the patient will listen with sympathy to her complaints and, as described in Chapter 8, his understanding of her condition and his choice of treatment will reflect his views on mental disease: if he adheres to the naturalistic tradition, he may institute behaviour therapy, or, more likely, he may choose to prescribe an anxiolytic drug.

Probably most doctors, even those who are particularly interested in biology, will have an uneasy feeling that there is something fundamentally wrong with these suggestions, especially the administration of drugs. The state of anxiety in this patient is an indication that she is desperately trying to give her life a new

Hermeneutics and the Nature of Man 123

meaning, and this existential problem is not just a biological dysfunction or inappropriate behaviour. We are dealing with a different dimension of life, and one may even suspect that effective drug treatment will diminish her chances of solving her problems.

We shall now try to discuss these vague ideas from a philosophical point of view and this is a difficult task. In the preceding chapters we have mentioned a number of philosophers, including Locke, Hume, Popper and Kuhn, but, in spite of the differences between their theories, they were all mostly concerned with the naturalistic tradition with which the modern scientifically minded doctor is well acquainted. In order to discuss the wider non-naturalistic concept of man, we must concern ourselves with so-called continental philosophy, which is linked to such names as Kierkegaard, Heidegger, Gadamer, Sartre and Habermas, and their ideas are much more difficult to grasp.

Continental philosophy is associated with terms like *existentialism, phenomenology* and *hermeneutics* (*hermeneutike* = art of interpretation), and to hint at the meaning of these words, one may say that these philosophers are concerned with the unique problem of human *existence* and that they approach this problem not by observation, but by philosophical reflection. They take an interest in the *phenomena* which are experienced by the human mind, and they seek to understand and *interpret* human action. In this brief presentation we shall concentrate on the thinking of the Danish philosopher Søren Kierkegaard (1813–55) and the German philosopher Martin Heidegger (1889–1976) who are important representatives of the non-naturalistic continental tradition. We shall ignore the diversity of this school of philosophy, which in this book will simply be labelled *the hermeneutic tradition*. The quotations from Kierkegaard and Heidegger on the next few pages will reveal that it is far beyond the scope of this book to discuss hermeneutic philosophy in any depth, and we only aim at giving the reader an impression of this very important, philosophical tradition. This chapter only serves as an introduction to the subsequent ones, in which we shall demonstrate the conflict between the purely naturalistic and the hermeneutic approaches to the solution of medical problems. In Chapters 10 and 11 we shall discuss the role of hermeneutic thinking in social medicine and psychiatry, in Chapters 12 and 13 we shall show that the concept of man in hermeneutic philosophy plays an important role in contemporary medical ethics, and in Chapter 14 we shall consider much more systematically the relationship between mind and body.

Anxiety as a fundamental state of mind

The following quotation from Kierkegaard illustrates well the non-naturalistic approach to the concept of anxiety or angst, as he asserts that this mood is not merely a psychiatric symptom, but a fundamental state of mind which cannot be eliminated:

> As the doctor will say that there is no man who is completely healthy, so you must say, if you know man well, that there is no human being alive who does not despair a little, who does not harbour an unrest, a discord, a disharmony, an angst of something unknown, of something with which he dares not acquaint himself, an angst of a possibility of life, or an angst of himself; so that he, as the doctor talks about having an illness of the body, also has an illness, has and sustains an illness of the spirit, which from time to time by glimpses reveals that it is here in the form of an angst which he cannot explain [2].

In order to understand the wider implications of this point of view, it is necessary to distinguish between constituent and contingent attributes. As an example, it is a constituent attribute of a cup that it is hollow so that it may be filled with a liquid, as it is simply impossible to imagine a cup which does not possess this property. In contrast, it is a contingent attribute of some cups that they are made of porcelain as it causes no logical difficulties to imagine a cup which is made of glass or metal. Thus, the elimination of the constituent qualities of an object or a phenomenon has the effect that it ceases to be an object or phenomenon of that particular kind, whereas the elimination of contingent attributes does not have this effect.

According to Kierkegaard, angst, despair and melancholy are constituent attributes of man, in just the same way as hollowness is a constituent attribute of a cup. Kierkegaard expresses the idea by stating that 'those human beings . . . whose soul knows no melancholy, are those whose soul senses no metamorphosis' [3]. Somebody who does not know melancholy or 'an angst of the potentiality of existence' is not a person; one of the constituent qualities of human nature is missing.

Since the renaissance, scientists have deepened our insight into the constitution of natural objects, like crystals, proteins, cells and tissues. They have gradually learnt to distinguish between those features which are essential and those which are not, and, as a result of this process, they have succeeded in establishing well-founded useful theories. As an example, biologists have rejected all forms of vitalism in their explanations of the functions of living organisms, as they claim that it has not yet proved possible to demonstrate any biological phenomenon which cannot be explained in terms of natural science.

Similarly, one may seek to determine the constituent features of man *as an individual who is able to act freely,* and not just as a particularly differentiated biological and social being. Those philosophers who belong to the hermeneutic tradition claim that the answer to such a problem cannot be found by empirical investigations, but must be sought by philosophical reflection. They try by introspection and reflection to determine those properties which as an ontological necessity constitute human nature.

Therefore, the hermeneutic inquiry is very different from the scientific one, but it is essential to note that philosophers, like Kierkegaard and Heidegger, do not deny that it is also important to study human beings empirically as is done in modern psychiatry and in modern medicine in general. Such studies, in which man is regarded as a biological and psychosocial being, serve to describe the actual situation in which an individual finds himself, and it is that situation which delimits his possibilities of action. However, as we shall discuss below, empirical data cannot be interpreted correctly, except in the light of hermeneutic reflection.

Phenomena like anxiety and depression are eminently well suited to illustrate the limitations of the naturalistic approach. From the hermeneutic point of view, anxiety is a constituent attribute of man, and it is a grave mistake always to regard it as something undesirable, or to conclude that severe anxiety is always a sign of disease. Anxiety is not primarily a pathological symptom, but, according to Heidegger, a state which permits 'privileged access to self-knowledge' [4]. That does not mean, of course, that anxiety is never a sign of disease, but those empirically minded psychiatrists who have chosen only to regard it as such, have committed themselves to a narrow and undifferentiated view of man. They overlook that basic moods, like anxiety, despair and depression, are as important for the possibilities of the personality as adrenalin for the function of the body.

It is the main theme of Kierkegaard's philosophy that man, as a self-reflecting free agent, is more than a biological and psychosocial synthesis, and he expresses this idea in the following quotation from *The Sickness Unto Death*. The passage is cryptic, but it is a good example of Kierkegaard's literary style, and it will be followed by an interpretation:

> Man is spirit. But what is spirit? Spirit is the self. But what is the self? The self is a relation which relates itself to its own self. ... Man is a synthesis of the indefinite and the finite, of the temporal and the eternal, of freedom and necessity, in short, a synthesis. A synthesis is a relation between two, the relation is the third as a negative unity ... such a relation is that between soul and body, when man is determined as soul. If, on the contrary, the relation relates itself to its own self, the relation is then the positive third, and this is the self [5].

The quotation is obviously not easy to understand, as it is written in an unusual style and refers to a particular philosophical discussion, but we shall try to explain the meaning in order to give a reasonably clear picture of Kierkegaard's theory of man, which is similar to that of other continental philosophers.

The first thing to note is that man is a synthesis of soul and body, of something mental and something physical. That part of the theory is little different from the view that man is a biological and psychosocial being, and therefore it is also in agreement with the holistic view in modern psychiatry, according to which illness is determined by a variety of interacting biological and psychosocial factors. The idea of a synthesis may well be interpreted as a multifactorial relationship, and to that extent Kierkegaard's theory encompasses modern naturalistic thinking.

However, if man was *no more* than this synthesis, if there was not a third element which united and completed the synthesis, human beings would be no different from animals. The third element, which determines that man is a person and not just a biological machine, is the spirit or the self. The self—or the personhood, as we say today—is the third element which constitutes man as man and determines his unique form of existence. We shall try to characterize this positive third a little further. In *The Sickness Unto Death* Kierkegaard also writes:

> The self is composed of infinity and finiteness. But the synthesis is a relationship, and it is a relationship which, though it is derived, relates itself to itself, which means freedom. The self is freedom [6].

He continues a little later:

> Altogether, consciousness, i.e. self-consciousness, is decisive in relation to the self. The more consciousness, the more self; the more consciousness, the more will; the more will, the more self. A man who has no will at all is no self; but the more will he has, the more self-consciousness does he also have.

That which unites the different elements of the human synthesis is the fact that man relates himself to himself and thereby understands himself as an individual who acts freely. The positive third is self-reflection and freedom.

Kierkegaard has presented his theory in the literary style of a bygone age, and the modern scientifically minded doctor may be reluctant to take seriously the idea that man is characterized by a 'self' or a 'positive third' which enables him to relate himself to himself. That, however, would be a great mistake.

Anybody who is trying to make a choice between different courses of action must be able to 'relate himself to himself' in the sense that he must be able to see himself in the situation in which he finds himself and in the possible developments of that situation. He is not only a conscious being with feelings, wishes and desires, but he is also a self-conscious being who is able to reflect on his own feelings, wishes and desires in relation to his self-chosen values and the conditions of his life.

Kierkegaard saw this clearly, and it is interesting that modern analytic philosophers have expressed much the same view. Thomas Nagel, for instance, writes in connection with a discussion about personal identity that each of us contains an objective self 'that has unlimited capacity to step back from the standpoint of the person I am in order to form a new conception of the world in which the person and his states are located' [7].

Human beings are characterized by their ability to understand

and interpret their actions and conditions in life, and a theory of man which aims at explaining the higher-level phenomena of human consciousness, e.g. the ability of man to choose in accordance with his own preferences, must by necessity take into account the 'self' or 'positive third'.

In summary, a human being may be characterized as a biological and psychosocial synthesis which is sustained by the self. It is the activity of the self, i.e. self-reflection, volition and free action, which regulates and harmonizes the interplay between biological and psychosocial factors. Natural scientists, who reduce self-reflection to something physical or to something mental or to a passive interaction between the two, are disregarding a constituent element of human beings. According to Kiekegaard, man without self is no longer human, and the self cannot be subsumed under biology or psychology. In psychiatry, these ideas have been developed further by those who regard psychoanalysis as a hermeneutic discipline, and we shall return to this topic in Chapter 11.

Now we shall resume the discussion of the concept of anxiety in the light of Kierkegaard's theory. He writes:

> The concept of angst is almost never considered in psychology, and I must therefore point out that it is quite different from fear and similar concepts which refer to something definite, while angst is the reality of freedom as a possibility for the possibility. Therefore, angst is not found in the animal, because by nature the animal is not determined by spirit [8].

Naturalistic psychiatrists only distinguish between mental and somatic phenomena, and they refer both rational fear and unexplained anxiety to the mind, but Kierkegaard's analysis goes further. He holds that man is a synthesis of a mind, a body and a self, and distinguishes sharply between feelings and fundamental moods. Angst—unexplained anxiety—which is an example of a fundamental mood, is uniquely human, as it is primarily associated with the self. It is a constituent feature of man as a self-reflective and freely acting individual, and it makes us realize 'the possibilities of freedom'. These possibilities at the same time attract and repel, and for that reason Kierkegaard has, somewhat cryptically, characterized angst as 'a sympathetic antipathy and an antipathetic sympathy' [8].

Rational fear, on the other hand, is a feeling, and, according to

Hermeneutics and the Nature of Man 129

Kierkegaard, feelings are purely mental phenomena. They are not dependent on self-reflection and freedom, and for that reason both animals and humans may experience fear when they are threatened.

In his important, but very difficult work *Being and Time* [4], Heidegger also analyses the concept of angst. He agrees with Kierkegaard that it is a basic mood, but adds that it is specifically linked to our understanding and interpretation of the world. In order to appreciate this idea, it must be pointed out that, according to Heidegger, 'understanding', like unexplained anxiety, is not a psychological phenomenon, but a constituent feature of human nature. 'Understanding' is what Heidegger calls an *existentiale*. The psychologist who says that we must try to understand the emotions, motives and actions of other people, regards 'understanding' as a specific psychological process, but Heidegger uses the word in a very different sense. For him, man is more than a biological organism which more or less passively responds to stimuli from outside; man is *qua* human being perpetually engaged in understanding—interpreting—the meaning of the world which faces him. Somebody who does not relate himself to the world as an understanding and interpreting human being has lost his subjectivity.

Angst is a mood which signifies that our previous understanding of the world has collapsed and that our contacts with other people have lost their meaning. We are, as Heidegger puts it, confronted with nothingness, and we are forced to mark out a new frame for the interpretation of our surroundings. It is in this sense that Heidegger characterizes angst as a state which permits privileged access to self-reflection: it points to the important dimension of human nature that we have the freedom to establish a new horizon of understanding and to see ourselves and the conditions of our life in a new light. Angst opens up new possibilities which at the same time attract and repel.

It follows from this discussion that, from a hermeneutic point of view, patients who suffer from unexplained anxiety must not only be treated in the medical sense; they must themselves come to grips with their problems, guided by self-reflection. The person who lives in a state of anxiety is free to choose, *must* choose, and he has also made a choice if he decides not to face the problems of his life, not to establish a new horizon of understanding, and chooses to relieve his anxiety by means of anxiolytic drugs. In that case, he has chosen to live an *unreal* life, as he has refused to provide his own answers to the problems of existence.

This discussion illustrates that differences of opinion regarding fundamental philosophical problems have practical consequences. Today, most people accept the naturalistic concept of man, and it is a logical consequence of that view that anxiolytic and antidepressant drugs have become a major commercial article all over the world. They have been tested in accordance with the most sophisticated scientific principles, and doctors prescribe them to their patients. Anxiety and depression are regarded as undesirable symptoms, just like toothache or a painful knee, and it is the doctor's duty, whenever possible, to eliminate unpleasant symptoms. Those who take the hermeneutic point of view seriously must question this aspect of our culture. As explained, they consider anxiety and depression to be constituent features of man as a person and, consequently, they must regard drug therapy, behaviour therapy or any other medical therapy as no less than a violation of the patient's integrity. Treatment with drugs must be limited to those conditions, e.g. delirium tremens, manic-depressive psychosis and schizophrenia, in which anxiety and depression are clearly pathological and not existential. Otherwise, drug treatment can only be defended, if it is clearly in accordance with the patient's own free choice.

Hermeneutics and natural science

Those who have been taught medicine, as if it was only a branch of natural science, must invariably wonder whether the assertions made by hermeneutic philosophers are true, and the answer which at least some empiricist philosophers provide to that question is quite clear: the assertions cannot be tested by scientific methods and, therefore, they are neither true nor false; they simply make no sense. Continental philosophers, of course, do not counter this argument by claiming that it is possible experimentally to prove the existence of 'the self', but they assert that the empiricists have not grasped the crux of the matter. They point out that natural science presupposes hermeneutic reflection; scientific experiments require that the scientist interprets and understands the problem under investigation, as it is the nature of that problem which determines his choice of method. The indiscriminate transfer of a scientific method from one area to another is impossible, even within the frame of conventional naturalistic thinking: a scientist can measure the renal function, but he cannot interview a kidney, and he can interview a person about his thoughts and intentions, but he cannot measure these mental activities. The empiricist who requires experimental proof of the existence of the self has forgotten to consider the constituent properties of a person, in much the same way as the scientist who endeavours to interview a kidney has not grasped the true nature of that organ. In other words, the hermeneutic analysis of the self is a prerequisite of empirical studies, as it makes no sense to study the properties of a particular person empirically, unless one has analysed the concept of a person. Therefore, natural science is subordinate to hermeneutic reflection.

It follows from this discussion that, according to the hermeneutic tradition, it is possible to ask meaningful questions which cannot be answered empirically, and a philosopher like Kierkegaard distinguishes sharply between objective and subjective reflection and between objective and subjective truth. Those who seek the objective truth only concern themselves with the subject-independent reality, and to them the relation between subject and object is of no relevance. In contrast, those who reflect subjectively cannot separate object from subject, as the subjective truth concerns the relationship between the two. The objective truth must be sought by methods of natural science, whereas the search for subjective truth requires the use of the hermeneutic method, i.e. interpretation and reflection [9].

The importance of subjective truths is well known in everyday medicine. In Chapter 4 the critic of the mechanical model of disease reported a number of case histories: a woman with asymptomatic arterial hypertension became distressed when her disease was diagnosed (p. 53); three duodenal ulcer patients interpreted their disease in very different ways; and the main source of the suffering of a woman with a metastasizing carcinoma was not the unpleasant symptoms, but her interpretation of her illness in relation to her own life (p. 56–7). In the context of the discussion in Chapter 4, these cases were used to demonstrate the limitations of the mechanical model of disease, but they also illustrate the clinical relevance of Kierkegaard's concept of human nature. What matters is not only the anatomical and physiological disturbances, but the way in which the patient relates herself or himself to the disease. What matters most is not the *objective truth,* but the *subjective truth* which is associated with 'the self' and differs from individual to individual.

Kierkegaard discusses this problem in general terms as he claims that the objective truth—objective reflection—is of little interest, when it is not related to the existence of the individual:

> The way of objective reflection makes the subject accidental, and thereby transforms existence into something indifferent, something vanishing. Away from the subject the objective way of reflection leads to the objective truth, and while the subject and his subjectivity become indifferent, the truth also becomes indifferent, and this indifference is precisely its objective validity; for all interest, like all decisiveness, is rooted in subjectivity. The way of objective reflection leads to abstract thought, to mathematics, to historical knowledge of different kinds; and it always leads away from the subject, whose existence or non-existence, and from the objective point of view quite rightly, becomes infinitely indifferent . . . [10].

Kierkegaard mentions mathematics and history, but he might just as well have mentioned modern medicine with its vast amount of empirical facts. The objective truths of scientific medicine are recorded in the 'language of abstraction', and they are only important when they are related to the existence of the individual patient.

Kierkegaard's attitude to the objective thinking of medical practitioners is well illustrated by the sarcasm of the following passage from *The Concept of Dread* in which he discusses angst in its most highly developed form which he calls 'the demoniacal':

> The demoniacal has been regarded therapeutically. It must, of course, be treated: *Mit Pulver und mit Pillen* [with powder and with pills]—and then clysters! Then the apothecary and the doctor put their heads together. The patient has been isolated so that others might not be afraid. In our courageous age one does not say to a patient that he will die, one does not dare to call the priest, for fear the patient might die of fright, one does

not dare to say to the patient that the same day a man died of the same illness. The patient was isolated, inquiries were made out of compassion, the physician promised to issue as soon as possible a tabulated statistical statement in order to determine the average. And when one has the average, everything is explained. The therapeutic point of view makes one regard the phenomenon as purely physical and somatic; one does as physicians often do, especially in Hoffmann's stories—one takes a pinch of snuff and says, 'This is a serious case' [11].

However, it must not be concluded from a passage like this one, as many mistakenly do, that hermeneutic philosophers, like Kierkegaard and Heidegger, deny the importance of natural science. They only insist that it must be seen in its proper perspective. Kierkegaard does not deny that angst—the demoniacal—may be regarded as a physical and somatic phenomenon; he only scorns the idea of some doctors that it is *purely* physical and somatic. In *The Concept of Dread* he points out that angst may also be viewed from other angles: it may be regarded as misfortune or fate which deserves compassion, or it may be regarded as something which deserves ethical condemnation. He concludes:

> The fact that such various ways of regarding it are possible shows how ambiguous is this phenomenon, and that in a way it belongs to all spheres, the somatic, the psychic and the pneumatic.* This indicates that the demoniacal covers a far greater field than is commonly supposed, and this can be explained by the fact that man is a synthesis of soul and body supported by the spirit, wherefore a disorganization in one shows itself in the others [11].

Heidegger in *Being and Time* arrives at much the same conclusion. He accepts 'that anxiety is often conditioned by "physiological factors"', but he also reminds us that only because this mood is a constituent feature of human nature 'does it become possible for anxiety to be elicited physiologically' [12].

These quotations show that the hermeneutic philosophers' theory of man does not ignore that man is a biological organism; they only point out that man as a person cannot be fully understood within a naturalistic frame. Those features which constitute man as

---
* i.e. pertaining to the spirit or the self.

a person, e.g. anxiety, freedom, will and understanding, cannot be analysed satisfactorily unless human nature is viewed in a wider perspective.

Notes and references

1 *Angst* is a German and Danish word which has become accepted in philosophical terminology. It is usually translated as 'dread' or 'anxiety'.
2 (a) Kierkegaard, S. *Sygdommen til Døden* (originally published 1849). In: Drachmann, A.B., Heiberg, J.L. & Lange, H.O. (eds) *Collected Works (Samlede Værker)*. Copenhagen: Gyldendal, 1963, vol. 15, p. 81. (b) English translation by W. Lowrie. *The Sickness unto Death*. London: Humphrey Milford, 1944, p. 32. The quoted passage has been translated by us.
3 (a) Kierkegaard, S. *Enten-Eller* (originally published in 1843). In: *Collected Works*, vol. 3, p. 178. (b) English translation by W. Lowrie. *Either/Or*. Princeton: Princeton University Press, 1944, p. 194.
4 (a) Heidegger, M. *Sein und Zeit* (originally published 1927). Tübingen: Max Niemeyer, 1976. (b) English translation by J. Macquarrie & E. Robinson. *Being and Time*. Oxford: Basil Blackwell, 1980, p. 228–35.
5 p. 73 in [2a] and p. 17 in [2b]. Lowrie's translation.
6 p. 87 in [2a] and p. 43 in [2b]. Lowrie's translation.
7 Nagel, T. The mind. In: McMurrin, S.M. (ed.) *The Tanner Lectures on Human Values 1980*, Cambridge: Cambridge University Press, 1980, p. 94.
8 (a) Kierkegaard, S. *Begrebet Angest* (originally published 1844). In: *Collected Works*, vol. 6, p. 136. (b) English translation by W. Lowrie. *The Concept of Dread*. Princeton: Princeton University Press, 1944, p. 38. Our translation.
9 In order not to oversimplify matters, it is important to add that the distinction between objective and subjective truth is not only the concern of hermeneutic philosophers; it is also considered a problem by contemporary analytic philosophers. We shall return to this topic in connection with the discussion of the mind–body problem in Chapter 14.
10 (a) Kierkegaard, S. *Afsluttende uvidenskabelig Efterskrift* (originally published 1846). In: *Collected Works*, vol. 9, p. 161. (b) English translation by D.F. Swenson & W. Lowrie. *Concluding Unscientific Postscript*. Princeton: Princeton University Press, 1944, p. 173. Swenson & Lowrie's translation.
11 p. 205 in [8a] and pp. 108–9 in [8b]. Partly based on Lowrie's translation.
12 p. 234 in [4b].

CHAPTER 10
MEDICINE AND SOCIOLOGY

*I*t has been known for a long time that the physical environment plays an important role in the development of disease. The observation that cholera epidemics are associated with the contamination of drinking water even predated the identification of the infective agent, and the fact that miners frequently develop lung disease could hardly go unnoticed in mining districts. Contemporary doctors have also learnt to appreciate that it is sometimes necessary to take into account social factors. Addiction to narcotics, for instance, is closely linked to certain urban subcultures, and the treatment of addicts requires considerations which cannot be contained within the biological concept of disease. Doctors can alleviate the withdrawal symptoms and they can even make the addicts stop taking drugs during prolonged confinement to institutions, but afterwards the patients must be resocialized. They must be offered jobs or education, and they must be motivated not to return to the milieu from which they came, but to seek new friends and a new purpose in life. Diseases like cholera, silicosis and drug addiction cannot be eliminated, unless we appreciate the importance of environmental and social factors.

Social medicine is now regarded as an independent medical discipline at most medical schools [1]. Sometimes it is even claimed that it is the only discipline which fully recognizes that a patient is not only a biological but also a social individual, and that sociomedical research is indispensable for the solution of major health problems of modern society. In this chapter we shall discuss the philosophical status of social medicine, which is of particular interest as we are concerned with the borderland between medicine and the social sciences.

First, we shall discuss the development of modern social medicine, which in many ways runs parallel to the development of other medical disciplines, and we shall be able to discern both realist and empiricist tendencies. Next, we shall take up the discussion from the preceding chapter and present the hermeneutic view of the social sciences, and we shall illustrate that the naturalistic and hermeneutic traditions represent two totally different concepts of man.

From classical epidemiology to empiricist social medicine

Modern social medicine originates from classical epidemiology. At first, epidemiologists were particularly interested in infectious diseases, and they framed what may be called the epidemiological model of disease, according to which the development of disease is seen as the result of an interaction between a pathogenic agent, environmental factors and a biological organism. Tuberculosis is a good example, as the spreading of that disease does not only depend upon the presence of the tubercle bacillus, but also on the living conditions of the population and the general state of health of its individual members. One must imagine a complex causal network, like the ones described in Chapter 5, and the difference between this model and the mechanical model used by clinicians is small. The clinician seeks the mechanical fault *inside* the body, whereas the epidemiologist is interested in the causes *outside* the body, but both are philosophical realists who imagine the existence of generative mechanisms which can be described in biological terms. It is, for instance, not difficult to explain that tuberculosis spreads more easily when people are living close together under poor housing conditions; there is a greater chance of droplet infection, and the bacilli survive better outside the human organism when it is dark and moist and when the standard of hygiene is low.

Later, the epidemiological model was extended in a number of respects, and, gradually, social medicine removed itself from classical epidemiology.

Firstly, the application of the epidemiological model is no longer restricted to infectious diseases, but is also used to analyse the causes of such diseases as cancer, arteriosclerosis and the so-called psychosomatic conditions. The medical sociologist may even use other disease criteria than those of the traditional disease classification; he may, for instance, study those people collectively who exhibit 'disease behaviour', e.g. consult their general practitioner or stay home from work for medical reasons.

Secondly, medical sociologists no longer restrict their attention to infectious agents and the physico-chemical characteristics of the environment; they also take into account the importance of such factors as social strata, subcultures, marital status and psycho-social events (life events), e.g. death of a relative, loss of a job or punishment for a criminal offence.

Thirdly, they do not only consider the biological characteristics of the probands (e.g. their ethnic origin or nutritional state), but also their personality and mental state. It may, for instance, be recorded whether people 'feel stressed', and it has been attempted to distinguish between different personality types and behaviour patterns by means of psychological tests. Recently, it has been claimed that myocardial infarction is associated with a particular behaviour pattern which is characterized by a high level of activity, restlessness and a competitive attitude to life [2].

Contemporary medical sociologists stress the importance of the extension of the classical epidemiological model, which in their opinion reflected a reductionist attitude to medicine. They claim that the development of the classical model into a *bio-psycho-social model* (see p. 117) was needed in order to replace biological reductionism by a *holistic* view of disease.

Socio-medical research workers use statistical methods in order to detect statistically significant correlations between different variables, and they hope that the resulting knowledge of causal relationships may prove helpful for the prevention of disease. We shall illustrate this analytical approach by means of a (fictitious) example.

At a factory the medical officer interviewed a sample of 300 workers, and 49 (16%) were found to suffer from an irritable bowel syndrome (constipation, abdominal discomfort, etc.). He also recorded that almost half of these workers did eight-hour

Table 3. Correlation between shift-work, stress and irritable bowel symptoms in 300 factory workers

Mode of work	Irritable bowel symptoms		
	Present (%)	Absent	Total
(a) All workers			
Shift-work	32 (23)	108	140
Day-work	17 (11)	143	160
Total	49 (16)	251	300
(b) Workers complaining of stress			
Shift-work	27 (39)	43	70
Day-work	9 (41)	13	22
Total	36 (39)	56	92
(c) Workers not complaining of stress			
Shift-work	5 (7)	65	70
Day-work	8 (6)	130	138
Total	13 (6)	195	208

shifts, whereas the remainder only worked during the day. These pieces of information were correlated, and it was discovered that the frequency of irritable bowel symptoms was twice as high among shift-workers as among day-workers (Table 3). The difference is so big that statistical testing will show that it is 'statistically significant'. However, the observation that some day-workers also suffered irritable bowel symptoms showed that shift-work was not the only cause, and more factors were included in the analysis. It had, for instance, also been recorded which workers had complained that they felt 'stressed' and, when this variable was taken into account, a different picture emerged (Table 3b and c). It is seen that irritable bowel symptoms occur much more frequently among those who feel stressed (39%) than among those who do not (6%), and the correlation between irritable bowel symptoms and mode of work disappears completely when the total sample is subdivided according to the presence or absence of stress. These results strongly suggest that the most important causal factor is stress and that shift-work only produces symptoms in so far as it produces stress [3].

This example of *analytical* socio-medical research was particularly simple, as it was possible to detect the causal relationship by simply looking at the figures, but many projects include so many variables that it is quite impossible to form a clear picture of the causal network by simple inspection. It is necessary to enter the results into a computer and to perform advanced multivariate statistical analyses in order to detect the hidden regularities.

Other medical sociologists concern themselves with *experimental* social medicine, and within that field the research methods are closely related to the ones which are used by those clinicians who belong to the critical clinical school (Chapters 1 and 3). Admittedly, the medical sociologist can rarely perform randomized controlled trials, but he can approach this ideal by using *quasi-experimental* designs [4]. In this connection it is interesting to note that the followers of the critical clinical school in the United States call themselves clinical epidemiologists, as they claim to have transferred the statistical approach from epidemiology to clinical medicine [5]. Some American medical schools have professors in clinical epidemiology, and they do not, as some might expect, concern themselves with population surveys, but with controlled therapeutic trials, the assessment of diagnostic tests, and statistical analyses of the causes of those diseases which are seen in hospital practice.

The development of the bio-psycho-social disease model from the epidemiological one has important philosophical implications. The epidemiologist, who thinks in terms of the classical model and, for instance, studies the association between air pollution and lung cancer, is a philosophical realist. He will do empirical studies and subject his results to a statistical analysis, but to him causality is more than a regular succession of events. If he finds a statistical correlation between the presence of a particular substance in the air and the occurrence of lung cancer, he is in no doubt that this substance generates the cancer by means of some mechanism or other. He will imagine that the substance is inhaled and that somehow it induces the malignant change in the bronchial epithelium.

The medical sociologist, however, does not think in this way. He prides himself that he also takes into account psychological and social factors, but the extension of the model has the unfortunate effect that it is much more difficult to think in terms of generative mechanisms. He may have found that the frequency of myocardial infarction is correlated to the socio-economic level or the feeling of stress, but the true nature of these variables differs from that of biological phenomena, and it is not unproblematic to state that a social factor, like affluence, or a mental state, like stress, generates myocardial infarction. Assertions of this kind require theories about the ontological status of social mechanisms, mental events and the interrelationship between the mind and the body. Some medical sociologists take little interest in such philosophical problems, and they may be characterized as extreme empiricists for whom the demonstration of statistical 'laws of nature' is regarded as the sole goal of science. The same empiricist tendency is found in some textbooks of sociological research methods. The authors discuss causality in full agreement with the succession theory [6] (see p. 19), stress the need for working definitions of social phenomena, suggest scoring systems for the measurement of such phenomena, and discuss statistical methods in great detail. But usually they ignore the fundamental philosophical problems.

It is also typical that some medical sociologists do not themselves see the schism between socio-medical research and traditional biological research, as it is one of the dogmas of empiricism that there is only *one scientific method*. The social sciences are regarded as less developed than natural science, but it is claimed that, in principle, there is no difference. Natural science makes use of sophisticated idealizations, like electrons, magnetic fields and neurotransmitters, whereas the social sciences, being less developed, use concepts like social strata and life events, which are much less precise. But the empiricists among social scientists still hope that they, just like natural scientists, will be able to demonstrate statistically significant correlations which may serve to predict future events. If it is found, for instance, that shift-work is often associated with irritable bowel symptons, it may be predicted that the abolition of shift-work will reduce the frequency of irritable bowel symptoms. This prediction does not presuppose any knowledge of the underlying mechanisms.

Criticism of empiricist sociology

The monoscientific ideal of the empiricists is by no means generally accepted by philosophers of science, and the use of the empirical methods of natural science for the explanation of social phenomena has been severely criticized. It has been asserted that there are two kinds of science: the natural sciences and the human or social sciences. The former are concerned with phenomena of nature which must be *explained* by demonstrating their causes, whereas the latter are concerned with human phenomena which must be *understood* in terms of the attitudes, feelings, norms and motives of the persons involved. Perhaps, it is possible by means of modern statistical methods to demonstrate significant correlations between alcoholism and a variety of social factors, and studies of that kind may explain the growth of alcoholism as the effect of, for instance, unemployment and changes in the pattern of family life; but the critics claim that the empiricist sociologist who confines himself to this kind of research does not come to grips with the real problems, as he does not take into account that the observed regularities are the result of the feelings, decisions and actions of individuals.

This criticism of empiricist sociology is associated with the school of thought which is called *methodological individualism*. Max Weber (1864–1920), who is one of the founders of modern sociology, thought along these lines, and, more recently, John Watkins (b. 1924) has expressed the idea as follows:

> Every complex social situation, institution or event is the result of a particular configuration of individuals, their dispositions, situations, beliefs, and physical resources and environment. There may be half-way explanations of large-scale social phenomena (say, inflation) in terms of other large-scale phenomena (say, full employment); but we shall not have arrived at rock-bottom explanations of such large-scale phenomena until we have deduced an account of them from statements about the dispositions, beliefs, resources and inter-relations of individuals [7].

It has also been claimed that the scientifically orientated sociologist, who cherishes the monoscientific ideal and thinks in terms of the bio-psycho-social model, regards man as a *passive* object, rather than an acting individual. In order to describe the observed correlations between social factors and different kinds of behaviour, he uses words like needs, drives and instincts—in much the same way as the physicist talks about the force of gravity and magnetic fields—and the resulting picture of man is that of an object which is fully controlled by inner and outer forces: there is little difference between human behaviour and the movements of a robot. It is, of course, commendable that attempts are made to explain those mechanisms which underlie the observed phenomena, but the empiricists among sociologists seem to forget that the language used for describing the mechanisms must somehow reflect the nature of the phenomena. The mechanisms in inanimate nature can be explained in terms of inner and outer forces, but social phenomena must be regarded as the product of *intentional action*. Harré and Secord, who have advocated a realist approach to both the natural and social sciences, write that 'it is only through reports of feelings, plans, intentions, beliefs, reason and so on that the meaning of social behaviour and the rules underlying social acts can be discovered' [8].

If, for instance, somebody asked us why we have written this chapter, we should not refer to the molecular movements in our brain cells or to abstract forces like our needs and instincts, but we should simply explain our *reasons:* we *decided* to write the chapter, as we *believed* that the fulfilment of this *plan* might induce the reader to *think about* these problems. As we shall discuss more fully in Chapter 14, the italicized words make little sense in the context of, say, physics and geology, but Harré and Secord believe that sociological theories can only be formulated in such *intentional language*. A concept of man which excludes the notion of intentional action is absurd.

It is not possible to discuss in detail the full spectrum of alternative sociological schools of thought. We have briefly mentioned the methodological individualism of, for instance, John Watkins and the realist approach which is advocated by Harré and Secord, but the remainder of this chapter will be devoted to a discussion of *hermeneutic sociology*. The three theories which we have selected for this discussion (analytical hermeneutics according to Peter Winch, Gadamer's hermeneutic theory and Habermas's critical theory) differ in a number of important respects, but they resemble each other in so far as their proponents agree that social phenomena must be understood and interpreted by means of a hermeneutic process and not only explained by the methods of natural science.

Analytical hermeneutics

In the preceding chapters we have written a little about the history of modern philosophy, and it is evident that a difference exists between the main trends of philosophical thinking in the English-speaking world and on the Continent of Europe. The empiricist tradition, with its emphasis on empirical facts and logical analysis, has been particularly strong in English-speaking countries, whereas many philosophers on the Continent have concerned themselves with metaphysical inquiries. We need only compare the philosophy of Locke and Hume (Chapter 2) with that of Kierkegaard and Heidegger (Chapter 9). Of course, we must not forget continental empiricists, like August Comte and the members of the important Vienna Circle, but on the whole continental philosophy is characterized by grand theory which has never been very popular in Britain and North America.

From this point of view, the ideas of the contemporary British philosopher, Peter Winch (b. 1926), are interesting. He is, like modern empiricists, interested in the problem of knowledge and the role of language, but his social theory in some respects resembles those of continental philosophers [9].

In his book *The Idea of a Social Science and its Relation to Philosophy* [10], Winch argues that many of the important theoretical issues which have been raised in the social sciences must be settled by *a priori* conceptual analysis, rather than by empirical research:

> For example, the question of what constitutes social behaviour is a demand for the elucidation of the *concept* of social behaviour. In dealing with questions of this sort there should be no question of 'waiting to see' what empirical research will show us; it is a matter of tracing the implications of the concepts we use [11].

The elucidation of fundamental concepts is of primary importance from an epistemological point of view, as 'our idea of what belongs to the realm of reality is given for us in the language we use. The concepts we have settle for us the form of the experience we have of the world' [12].

Winch argues that our conception of reality depends upon the language we use and that our language is inextricably bound up with our way of living. Therefore, there are very close ties between epistemology (p. 14), language and social theory.

These ideas are to a large extent based on Ludwig Wittgenstein's linguistic philosophy, as it is expressed in his later work *Philosophical Investigations* [13]. Wittgenstein holds that our language and our way of living are inseparably bound up with one another, in the sense that our language is constituted by our way of living, just as our way of living is constituted by our language. This thesis can be illustrated by a concept, like a *promise*. The person who says, 'I promise to come tomorrow' has, if he is honest, entered into a social contract. The content of the word *promise* is linked to a particular social institution, according to which people may bind each other by means of promises and obligations. In the absence of such an institution the word has no meaning. Conversely, the existence of this social institution depends on language, as the persons involved must be able to communicate to each other that they are making promises or accepting obligations.

The making of a promise is a conscious, intentional act, and, as illustrated by this example, intentional action requires social institutions and generally accepted rules of conduct. Wittgenstein goes so far as to claim that language itself is a social institution and that those who speak a natural language perform particular acts— speech acts—in accordance with the rules of that language. The use of language and intentional action cannot be separated, as one is a precondition of the other.

The most fundamental social institution in any social setting is the implicit acceptance of the rules of language. People who are living together—who are enjoying a certain form of life— sometimes agree and sometimes disagree, but they can only express their agreement or disagreement in the language which is a constitutive part of that form of life. In Wittgenstein's words: 'It is what human beings *say* that is true or false; and they agree in the language they use. That is not agreement in opinions but in form of life' [14].

Winch draws the conclusion from those considerations that it is impossible to explain social behaviour in a cultural setting, unless one understands the social institutions and the language of that particular culture or subculture:

'A psychoanalyst who wished to give an account of the aetiology of neuroses amongst, say, the Trobriand Islanders, could not just apply without further reflection the concepts developed by Freud for situations arising in our own society. He would first have to investigate such things as the idea of fatherhood amongst the islanders and take into account any relevant aspects in which their idea differed from that current in his own society' [15].

In the same way, the medical sociologist, who concerns himself with the use of marijuana and other 'mood expanders' by members of certain subcultures, must acquire an understanding of their form of life, including their attitudes, values and language. Without such insight their actions may seem totally irrational. Of course, he may confine himself to a description of their behaviour, but the detection of regular behaviour patterns permits no understanding of the underlying 'mechanisms' which take the form of obligations and expectations that are communicated and sustained by the particular language of the subculture.

The sociologist seeks an unreflective understanding of the culture or subculture he is investigating, be it the Trobriand Islanders or marijuana users; he tries to understand their form of life as they understand it themselves, but he will also want to see the results of his studies in a wider theoretical perspective. For that purpose he may use technical terms which would be quite incomprehensible to the people he was studying, but, according to Winch, these theoretical concepts must be logically tied to the activities under investigation. Theoretical explanations in the social sciences presuppose the unreflective kind of understanding.

It is obvious from this presentation that *understanding* is a key concept in analytical hermeneutics, and it is important to note that the understanding of meaningful behaviour, which is the goal of the hermeneutic analysis, is not, as claimed by many empiricists, something private and subjective. The medical sociologist does not understand the marijuana user in the sense that he sympathizes with him or 'shares his feelings'; he is not concerned with feelings at all, but with *knowledge*. He wants to know as much as possible about the rules of behaviour, including the rules of language, of that particular subculture, and he will say that he understands the form of life of that person when the sum of his knowledge forms a meaningful whole. Such knowledge can be communicated to others by means of language, and for that reason it is not, as claimed by empiricists, private and subjective; it is *public and inter-subjective*. According to this view of the hermeneutic process, it is possible to distinguish between understanding and misunderstanding in much the same way as it is possible to ascertain whether a student of a foreign language has understood or misunderstood a particular word. As we shall see, other philosophers disagree on this.

German hermeneutic social theory

We shall now shift our attention from Britain to Germany, which is the home of hermeneutic philosophy. We have already introduced Heidegger (Chapter 9), and we shall now briefly consider the contributions of Heidegger's pupil, Hans-Georg Gadamer (b. 1900), who has taken a particular interest in the application of hermeneutic thinking to the humanities and the social sciences.

As already mentioned, analytical hermeneutics is based on Wittgenstein's theory, which aims at explaining what it means to master a language and to participate in a form of life, and, according to which, the process of understanding is likened to the process of learning a foreign language. Gadamar, however, does not accept this point of view: '... the hermeneutic problem is not one of the correct mastery of language, but of the proper understanding of that which takes place through the medium of language' [16].

Originally, the word hermeneutics was used in the sense 'biblical interpretation', i.e. the search for the spiritual truth in the Bible, and we may illustrate the conventional view of the hermeneutic process by imagining someone who is trying to understand a difficult literary text. He seeks to understand the text from the author's point of view, and he has succeeded in this task, if he has managed to reproduce the meaning of the text, as it was intended by the author. The sociologist who is studying an alien culture acts in a similar manner. He endeavours to grasp the intrinsic rationality of the behaviour of the participants in that culture, and in the course of the process he excludes his own prejudices, attitudes and opinions.

From Gadamer's point of view, this description of the hermeneutic process is totally wrong, as he believes that the problem of understanding only arises in the form of a confrontation between two 'forms of life', or to use his own expression, two *horizons of understanding*. He denies that those who attempt to understand a literary text, a work of art or the behaviour of a drug user can possibly exclude their own pre-understanding and prejudices [17].

Let us look at the process which leads to the understanding of a difficult text, this time from Gadamer's point of view. The student reads the text, which 'speaks to him' from the author's horizon of knowledge, attitudes, prejudices, etc., and, on the basis of his own horizon of understanding, he forms an incomplete picture of the meaning of the text. He then 'puts questions' to the text, and the 'answers' help him to improve the provisional interpretation. In this way the hermeneutic process takes the form of a 'dialogue' between the student and the author, and through this dialogue the student gradually attains a deeper understanding of the meaning. This process, which is often called the *hermeneutic circle,* only comes to an end when full agreement has been attained between the interpretation of the elements of the text (words, sentences and paragraphs) and the interpretation of the text as a whole. Gadamer uses the expression that at this stage the horizons of the interpreter and the author have fused, and this formulation has two very important implications.

Firstly, it is implied that the end-result of the hermeneutic process is not simply a reproduction of the intentions of the author when he wrote the text. The final interpretation also incorporates the interpreter's pre-understanding, and another interpreter with a different background would by necessity have understood the text differently. Thus, according to Gadamer, the interpretation of a text is subjective, as it depends on the interpreter, but it is not private as it can be formulated in language and communicated to others.

Secondly, the fusion of the horizons implies that the interpreter has incorporated something of the meaning of the text into his own life. The outcome of the hermeneutic process is not just that the interpreter has learnt to understand that particular text, but also that his own horizon of understanding has changed.

Gadamer's ideas apply even better to a dialogue between two people. A medical sociologist who wishes to understand somebody who uses 'psychedelic' drugs, i.e. LSD and mescalin, must acquaint himself with that person's language and life style. Therefore, they must engage in a dialogue which requires openness and frankness from both of them. Gadamer writes:

> ... it is characteristic of every true conversation that each opens himself to the other person, truly accepts his point of view as worthy of consideration and gets inside the other to such an extent that he understands not a particular individual, but what he says [18].

On the basis of his own pre-understanding, the sociologist forms a preliminary picture of the drug user's life style and way of thinking, and during the subsequent exchange, which is needed to revise and complete that picture, both parties will disclose their horizons. Ideally, they will learn to know each other so well that their horizons of understanding fuse, and in that case they will, both of them, have learnt something from the life style of the other.

In order to illustrate this idea, we shall recall the situation in the 1960s when the popularity of psychedelic drugs in some urban subcultures was at its peak. The first impression of a doctor or a sociologist might well have been that the use of these dangerous drugs was totally irrational, but an open dialogue with members of the subculture would have revealed that this was not the case. On the contrary, many of these people had a good grasp of their own situation, and they might even have pitied the doctor who had not had the same emotional experiences, but had devoted himself to his career rather than to the enjoyment of life. Under those circumstances the doctor would have been forced to see his own life in a new perspective, and he would also have had to appreciate that it was not sufficient to tell the young people that the drugs were dangerous. Effective 'treatment' would have required that, through his openness, he would have succeeded in making them accept something of his view of life and some of his values.

Gadamer is concerned with the historical dimension of the hermeneutic process. The philosophy of Wittgenstein and Winch is ahistorical in the sense that historical tradition plays no major role in their theories, but Gadamer claims that our understanding of a form of life or a text always reflects our position in a historical tradition. There is no such thing as understanding without pre-understanding, and our pre-understanding is shaped by the cultural tradition to which we belong. We cannot understand anything except in a historical perspective.

Tradition also plays the important role that it may help us to distinguish between true understanding and misunderstanding. As explained, no objective criteria exist by means of which we may assess whether our understanding is true or whether it is thwarted by false pre-understanding, and Gadamer believes that the truth can only emerge, if we view our understanding in a historical perspective:

> It is only this temporal distance that can solve the really critical question of hermeneutics, namely of distinguishing the true prejudices, by which we understand, from the false one by which we misunderstand. Hence the hermeneutically trained mind will also include historical consciousness [19].

As we shall explain below, Jürgen Habermas disagrees strongly with Gadamer on this point.

Critical theory

The German philosopher Jürgen Habermas (b. 1929) belongs to the so-called Frankfurt School, which originally was associated with the Institute for Social Research at the University of Frankfurt am Main. This philosophical school, which is based on Karl Marx's early writings, opposes both empiricism (p. 15) and dogmatic Marxism. Habermas's theories are in many ways problematic and not always clear, but they have played a major role in the contemporary debate on the status of the social sciences, and here we shall discuss some of his ideas, as they were expressed in his book *Knowledge and Human Interests* [20].

Habermas claimed that Gadamer's description of the hermeneutic process does not provide sufficient guarantee that our understanding of social relations is not distorted by false pre-understanding. It is not sufficient that the sociologist openly and frankly, through a hermeneutic circle, tries to understand a particular form of life. Society is characterized by its power structure and by clashes of interests which colour our understanding of ourselves and others, and mere 'historical consciousness' is not sufficient to prevent the sociologist's understanding from being *ideologically* distorted.

Ideology is a key concept in Habermas's philosophy, and it is used in a very special sense. An ideology is not any theory or set of beliefs, but a theory which serves the interests of particular groups in society and helps to cement existing power relations. It is a set of beliefs which has a repressive effect and provides a distorted view of reality. Ideological distortions may occur, when a word or a concept which was developed in one particular context is used in others where it does not belong. There is, for instance, a big difference between *treating* a case of pneumonia with penicillin and *treating* a political dissenter with tranquilizers and sedatives. The first example is ideologically neutral, whereas the second is ideologically distorted. In the latter case the word *treat* is used as part of the legitimation of a particular political power structure, and those who have been indoctrinated into believing that political dissent is a 'disease' which requires medical treatment, possess what in Habermas's terminology is called false consciousness. This example is, of course, particularly crude, but Habermas believes that more or less subtle ideological distortions imbue the understanding, attitudes and views of all of us to such an extent that it affects all communication among men. One might, for instance, discuss whether the idea, that alcoholism and neuroses are diseases in need of treatment, is ideologically neutral [21].

Therefore, the establishment of ideologically neutral social theories requires that the hermeneutic approach be supplemented with a critical analysis, which has a number of components. The most important of these is *ideology critique,* which directly serves to uncover the ideological distortions, but it is also necessary to do empirical studies of the structure of society and to analyse its historical development [22].

In *Knowledge and Human Interests*, Habermas develops his social theory. Basically, it is an anthropological one, as it is founded on an analysis of the characteristics of man. He stresses that man is a social being and distinguishes between two kinds of social activity, *work* and *interaction,* which are responsible for man's historical development.

Medicine and Sociology   151

According to Habermas, work and interaction imply the *fundamental interests of man*. Human beings are characterized by their *technical interest*, as they have to work, i.e. to perform purposeful, instrumental action in order to ensure their survival and reproduction. They must produce tools in order to procure food and they must produce clothes in order to protect themselves against cold. They are also characterized by the *practical or hermeneutical* interest, as it is equally important for the development of the human species that its members are able to interact with one another. They must develop a language in order to communicate and to understand each other, and they must establish social institutions. Finally, man is characterized by the *emancipatory interest*, which we shall discuss below.

It is evident from this presentation that fundamental human interests in Habermas's theory are not subjective interests. They are not interests in the usual sense of the word, but those motive forces which, in accordance with man's nature, determine his development. Habermas writes: 'I term *interests* the basic orientations rooted in specific fundamental conditions of the possible reproduction and self-constitution of the human species, namely work and interaction' [23].

Different kinds of scientific activity are governed by different interests. Natural science and technology are associated with the *technical interest*, and the achievements in these areas may be seen as the result of a continuous process which started when man first learnt to handle and produce simple tools. Through our scientific activities we acquire knowledge of our environment and we learn to exploit inanimate nature. In a similar manner, we study the structure and functions of living organisms, and biological medicine, which aims at the treatment and prevention of biological dysfunction, must also be referred to the technical interest. Habermas fully recognizes the importance of natural science, but he strongly opposes the so-called *scientistic misunderstanding* that knowledge can only be acquired by means of the methods of natural science. Therefore, Habermas would not deny the necessity of empirical studies in social medicine, provided we remember that this approach only serves the technical interest.

The *practical or hermeneutic interest* has determined the development of linguistic and symbolic communication among people and, on the scientific level, this interest is associated with the human or cultural sciences, typically sociology, psychology, linguistics and history. As mentioned above, empirical studies also play an important role in these disciplines, but the understanding and interpretation of the phenomena belong to the domain of hermeneutics.

Habermas describes the importance of these sciences in the following way:

> It [hermeneutic understanding] bans the dangers of communication breakdown in both dimensions: the vertical one of one's own individual life history and the collective tradition to which one belongs, and the horizontal one of mediating between the traditions of different individuals, groups, and cultures. When these communication flows break off and the intersubjectivity of mutual understanding is either rigidified or falls apart, a condition of survival is disturbed, one that is as elementary as the complementary condition of the success of instrumental action: namely the possibility of unconstrained agreement and non-violent recognition. Because this is the presupposition of practice, we *call the knowledge-constitutive interest of the cultural sciences 'practical'* [24].

The *emancipatory or critical interest* is not associated with any of the known sciences, except perhaps philosophy, but, according to Habermas, it is the interest which governs what he calls *critical science,* and, as discussed at the beginning of the chapter, the most important method of this kind of scientific activity is ideology critique.

From a medical point of view, it is particularly interesting that Habermas regards psychoanalysis as an example of 'critical science'. As we shall explain in the next chapter, psychoanalysis is primarily a hermeneutic discipline, as it serves to make the patients understand those unconscious psychological mechanisms which may explain their neurotic inhibitions, but attainment of such understanding is not the real purpose. The aim of psychoanalysis is therapeutic, as it is claimed that the insight into the causes of the psychological problem will *emancipate* the patients from those inhibitions which limit their social activity. Habermas, like Erich Fromm before him [25], draws an analogy between the neurosis of the individual patient and the state of society. In the same way as the patient's problem reflects unconscious psychological conflicts, the problems of society reflect unarticulated conflicts of interests, and it is hoped that ideology critique, just like psychoanalysis, may serve to dissolve unacceptable repressive structures. For this reason, the critical interest is also said to be emancipatory.

Critical theory as a whole may be regarded as an attempt to develop a comprehensive social theory which takes into account our need to exploit the resources of nature for our own purpose, our need to communicate with others, and our need to free ourselves from those constraints which are imposed upon us by repressive mechanisms in society.

The theory also shows that we may approach the study of society in a number of ways and that each method has its own meaningful but limited sphere of application. Empirical investigations are important, as they serve to describe social phenomena; hermeneutic studies are equally important, as they enable us to understand these phenomena; and ideology critique is needed to ensure that social theories do not only serve to confirm particular interests and to sustain the existing power structure.

Habermas's attempt to integrate radically different methods for the study of social and human phenomena is inspiring, but the correspondence between the three fundamental human interests and different kinds of science may not be quite as close as he wishes us to believe. The correspondence, for instance, between natural science and the technical interest can only be defended, if natural science is identified with empirical research on the technological level. However, as pointed out in Chapter 3, a distinction must be made between 'basic' science and technology, and it is not certain that the generation of new theoretical knowledge by means of basic research only serves a technical purpose. Habermas also takes it for granted that the hermeneutic method is the only one which can be used for the study of attitudes, motives, purposes and other intentional phenomena, but that is equally uncertain. It has, for instance, been suggested by Harré and Secord (p. 142) that the realist aproach to natural science may also be applicable to the study of social and human phenomena, if the theories are formulated in intentional language. Habermas's anthropological views, which form the basis of his theory, are also in dispute [26].

In spite of these criticisms, we shall accept that man has technical, hermeneutic and critical interests, and Habermas has correctly demonstrated some of the deficiencies of empiricist thinking. His theory may not be tenable in its present form [26], but the message which it conveys is of considerable interest to all sociologists, including the medical ones.

Thus, Habermas's theory can easily be applied to social medicine which concerns all these interests. Up to now, the empiricist approach to socio-medical problems has been the dominant one, and for that reason social medicine has mainly served the technical interest. Usually, medical sociologists confine themselves to studying the statistical correlation between more or less well-defined social variables, and they show little interest in the mechanisms which underlie these regularities. Such studies may contribute important factual information, but they cannot provide more than a rudimentary understanding of social relations. They may form the basis of administrative measures, but they do not ensure that these measures are desirable or legitimate.

In the human sciences attempts have been made to develop hermeneutic methods which permit systematic studies of motives, norms, values and attitudes, and these concepts are crucial for understanding social interaction. Medical sociologists must also adopt these hermeneutic methods, if they regard social medicine as more than a social technology and hope to contribute to the understanding of health problems.

Finally, it must be remembered that the attitude in society to socio-medical problems is invariably coloured by the spectrum of interests and the distribution of power in that society. Therefore, it is possible that empirical and hermeneutic studies ought to be supplemented with 'critical' socio-medical research.

Notes and references

1 We are referring to the fact that most medical schools have a chair in social medicine, epidemiology, community medicine or public health. Here we do not distinguish between these disciplines and, for the purpose of the discussion in this book, we have chosen the first of the terms. In Scandinavia a person who is engaged in socio-medical research, or who practises social medicine, is called a *socialmediciner* (a social physician), but in English no such word exists. We have chosen the term *medical sociologist,* which is supposed to comprise doctors concerned with the social aspects of medicine as well as sociologists who concern themselves with health problems.
2 A review panel. Coronary-prone behaviour and coronary heart disease: a critical review. *Circulation,* 1981; 63: 1199–215.
3 In order not to mislead the reader, we shall mention that, to our knowledge, it

has never been shown that stress produces irritable bowel symptoms. It is, however, well established that the occurrence of functional gastrointestinal complaints is related to shift-work (Andersen, J.E. *Three-shift work. A Socio-Medical Survey*. Danish National Institute of Social Research. Copenhagen: Teknisk Forlag, 1970).

4 The medical sociologist may, for instance, do a non-randomized controlled study in which he compares a group of persons, who are exposed to a certain environmental factor, to a control group of unexposed persons, who are comparable in all those respects which are known to be relevant. He may also use a time series design, which means that he carries out repeated observations on the same persons and then relates the results to the occurrence of a particular exposition.

5 The term *clinical epidemiology* was originally introduced by A. R. Feinstein (Yale University). Recently, the following textbook has appeared: Fletcher, R.H., Fletcher, S.W. & Wagner, E.H. *Clinical Epidemiology—the Essentials*. Baltimore: Williams and Wilkins, 1982.

6 e.g. Selltiz, C., Jahoda, M,. Deutsch, M. & Cook, S.W. *Research Methods in Social Relations*. London: Methuen, 1971.

7 Watkins, J.W.N. Ideal types and historical explanations. *British Journal for the Philosophy of Science*, 1952; 3: 29ff.

8 Harré, R. & Secord, P.F. *The Explanation of Social Behaviour*. Oxford: Basil Blackwell, 1972.

9 We have chosen Winch's theory as an example of analytical hermeneutics, i.e. theories concerning the problems of inter-subjective understanding, which are based on a formal or logical analysis. G. H. von Wright also represents this school of thought.

10 Winch, P. *The Idea of a Social Science and its Relation to Philosophy*. London: Routledge & Kegan Paul, 1958.

11 p. 18 in [10].

12 p. 15 in [10].

13 Wittgenstein, L. *Philosophical Investigations*. Oxford. Basil Blackwell, 1953.

14 p. 88 (§241) in [13].

15 p. 90 in [10].

16 Gadamer, H.-G. *Wahrheit und Methode*, 2nd edn. Tübingen: J.C.B. Mohr, 1965 (English translation by Glen-Doepel, W. *Truth and Method*, 2nd edn. London: Sheed & Ward, 1979, pp. 346–7).

17 Prejudice is translated from *Vorurteil*, and the word is used in its neutral sense (pre-judgment).

18 p. 347 in [16].

19 p. 266 in [16].

20 Habermas, J. *Erkenntnis und Interesse*. Frankfurt am Main: Suhrkamp, 1968 (English translation by Shapiro, J.J. *Knowledge and Human Interests*. London: Heinemann, 1972). Habermas is difficult to read and the presentation of his theory in the following book is more accessible: McCarthy, T. *The Critical Theory of Jürgen Habermas*. London: Hutchinson, 1978.

21 Habermas explains this idea as follows: 'Language is *also* a medium of domination and social power. It serves to legitimate relations of organized force. In so far as the legitimations do not articulate the relations of force that they

make possible, in so far as these relations are merely expressed in the legitimations, language is also ideological. Here it is not a question of deceptions within a language, but of deception with language as such. Hermeneutic experience that encounters this dependency of the symbolic framework on actual conditions changes into the critique of ideology'. Quoted from McCarthy [20], p. 183.
22 For Habermas, historical materialism constitutes the philosophical basis of historical studies. In classical Marxism it is the theory that the evolution of mankind is the product of the forces and relations of production, but, as explained on p. 151, Habermas has replaced these concepts by those of work and interaction.
23 p. 196 in [20], English edition.
24 p. 176 in [20], English edition.
25 Fromm, E. *The Sane Society*. London: Routledge and Kegan Paul, 1956.
26 The following book contains a number of important, critical papers: Thompson, J.B. & Held, D. (eds) *Habermas. Critical Debates*. London: Macmillan, 1982. In one of the papers ('A reply to my critics') Habermas himself writes that his works 'are at best stimulating, but by no means present finished thoughts'.

CHAPTER 11
PSYCHOANALYSIS: NATURAL SCIENCE OR HERMENEUTICS?

*I*n the preceding two chapters some of the main themes of hermeneutic philosophy were introduced, and earlier in this book it was pointed out that hermeneutic thinking is also important in somatic medicine. We discussed a number of cases (of duodenal ulcer disease, asymptomatic hypertension and metastasizing carcinoma), and it was concluded (Chapter 4) that the clinician must take into account not only the anatomical and physiological abnormalities, but also the meaning which the patient attaches to the disease and its symptoms in the context of his or her own life.

In this chapter we shall once again consider psychiatry, which is the medical discipline that constitutes the true battleground between hermeneutic and naturalistic thinking. In particular, we shall discuss the philosophical status of psychoanalysis, which was introduced as a scientific method but later evoked scathing criticism both from biologically orientated psychiatrists and from philosophers of science belonging to the empiricist tradition.

Freudian psychoanalysis

The psychoanalytical theory which was developed by Sigmund Freud (1856–1939) has had such an influence that today it has to some degree been incorporated into our culture. Therefore, we shall not discuss this theory in great detail, but we shall only, as a continuation of the discussion in Chapter 9, present briefly the psychoanalytical view of the concept of anxiety. The American psychiatrist Cameron gives this account:

Psychoanalytic theories regard anxiety as a symptom of an emerging repressed conflict, which is unacceptable to the rational-conscious part of the personality ('the ego'), and which is derived from the interplay between three different parts of the psychic apparatus, the 'superego, the ego and the id'. The threatened breakthrough of the repressed material is manifested as anxiety, and alerts the ego to take defensive action. If the defences are successful, the anxiety is contained, if not, important symptoms in neuroses and psychoses appear, resulting in either a partly or an almost complete disintegration of the ego. The manner in which anxiety, a major factor in structuring early personality development, is defended against is thus of utmost importance with respect to the personality structure of a person, justifying the claim, that anxiety is the cornerstone of all psychopathology [1].

In this way, the psychoanalyst regards symptoms like anxiety or phobias as the result of a complex interplay between the mental functions which Freud called the superego, the id and the ego. Somewhat simplified, the *superego* may be characterized as that part of the personality which is concerned with moral judgment. It is the person's conscience and it contains a system of norms, values and ideals, which have been absorbed from the traditions of the family and the surrounding society. The *id* represents the inborn primitive instincts of man, especially those which are related to sex and aggression, i.e. those processes which aim at immediate satisfaction by the enhancement of pleasure and the reduction of pain. The *ego* is the executive part of the personality which faces up to the demands of the real world and regulates both the impulses of the id and the constraints of the superego. Whereas the id is governed by the pleasure principle, the ego is governed by the reality principle.

Freud also introduced many other abstract concepts in his attempt to establish the structure of the personality and to explain its development, and the psychoanalyst uses this set of concepts when he tries to interpret what his patient tells him. The patient's symptoms may at first seem wholly inappropriate and irrational, and it is one of the purposes of psychoanalysis to uncover the structure and function of the patient's personality to such an extent that the symptoms are at last seen in a meaningful context. To reach this end it may be necessary to analyse not only the interaction between analyst and patient, but also dreams and slips of the tongue. It is believed that the process of working through the unconscious conflicts and the resulting insight may induce that enduring change of the personality which is regarded as cure.

A single Freudian example may help to illustrate these ideas. A young woman suffered from the phobia that she dared not touch objects which were made of rubber. She had had this phobia for as long as she could remember, but she did not know its cause. Psychoanalysis made her remember that, once when she was a small girl, her father had bought two balloons, one for herself and one for her sister. In a fit of bad temper she destroyed her sister's balloon and she was severely punished by her father. The analysis revealed that she had been very jealous of her smaller sister, so much that she had secretly wished that her sister would die so that she could be the sole object of her father's affection. The destruction of the balloon was a destructive action directed against her sister, and, consequently, the punishment and her own sense of guilt became associated with the rubber balloon. Each time she happened to touch rubber, her old fear of destroying her sister made her shrink away [2]. In this way, the psychoanalysis revealed that the seemingly irrational fear of rubber could be interpreted in terms of an unconscious conflict between a primitive id-function and the constraint imposed upon her by the superego.

This presentation must not give the impression that psychoanalysis is a single well-defined theory of psychopathology. Freud, himself, gradually changed his theory, and his thoughts have later been developed and greatly modified by many others. Therefore, many psychiatrists prefer the term psychodynamic theories which comprise both the original Freudian school and the separate streams of psychotherapy which developed later in different parts of the world. Carl Jung in Switzerland and Alfred Adler in Austria developed psychodynamic theories of their own; Anna Freud (Freud's daughter) and Melanie Klein, who both settled in Britain, may be regarded as the founders of psychoanalysis in children. Other analysts who also left Germany and Austria in the 1920s and 1930s established themselves in the United States, where they found a health service based on private enterprise and an individualistic attitude which provided good opportunities for psychoanalytical practice. The psychoanalytical tradition in this way gained a strong foothold in American psychiatry, and its further development is associated with such names as Hartmann, Sullivan, Karen Horney, Erikson and Rapaport.

In Europe, opinions were more divided, and psychoanalysis has been strongly criticized from different quarters. In his famous book *General Psychopathology,* published in 1913, the psychiatrist and existentialist philosopher, Karl Jaspers, characterized Freudianism as 'a movement of faith within the guise of science', and he considered psychoanalysis a danger from a philosophical point of view, as it was a kind of sect, tending to 'nihilism, a callous fanaticism and an arbitrary philosophical scepticism' [3]. Most critics, however, belong to the empiricist and biological traditions of psychiatry, which have dominated especially British and Scandinavian psychiatry, and we shall consider their criticism more closely.

Psychoanalysis as science

It is obvious that psychoanalysis differs dramatically from the scientific theory formation which characterizes biological medicine, but there can be no doubt that Freud saw himself as a natural scientist engaged in determining the structure of the mental apparatus. This attitude to psychoanalysis has also dominated American psychiatry, and Hartmann, to a greater extent that anybody else, has argued that psychoanalysis is a scientific theory about mental phenomena, and that analysts, just like 'other' natural scientists, seek causal explanations [4]. Hence, psychoanalytical theory was framed in such a way that the mind was conceived almost as a mechanical model which functions by 'hydraulic principles' under the influence of the ego, the id and the superego.

However, those who maintain that psychoanalysis is a kind of natural science are vulnerable to the criticism that it is impossible to test whether their theories are true. A scientist who postulates that the adrenal cortex produces a particular hormone, and that the size of the production is regulated by a feedback mechanism which involves the pituitary gland, will be able to test this theory by means of physiological experiments, but it is impossible even to suggest an experiment which may prove or disprove the existence of the superego or the importance of unconscious sexual impulses. It is

Psychoanalysis: Natural Science or Hermeneutics? 161

also impossible to test the truth value of psychoanalytical interpretations in the individual case, and the scientists among doctors will not feel quite convinced that the woman's fear of rubber was in fact caused by her jealousy towards her sister, and they will be even more sceptical when Freud interprets a dream in this way: 'The male genital organ is represented by three persons, the female by a landscape with a church, a mountain and a wood. Once again you see a stair as a symbol of the sexual act' [5].

It is surprising that Freud seems to have taken no interest in the testability problem. Once, when he was shown the results of an empirical study which seemed to support his theory, he is reported to have said:

> I have examined your experimental studies for the verification of the psychoanalytic assertions with interest. I cannot put much value on these confirmations because the wealth of reliable observations on which these assertions rest make them independent of experimental verification. Still, it can do no harm [6].

This quotation illustrates that psychoanalysts do not take the testability problem seriously, but feel convinced that their theories are true, simply because they are confirmed again and again by their patients. This way of thinking has been sharply criticized by Karl Popper, who maintains that the idle collection of more and more confirmatory instances never serves to prove the truth of a scientific theory. In *Conjectures and Refutations,* Popper mentions psychoanalysis as a particularly glaring example of this mode of thought, and with vitriolic sarcasm he recounts the following incident:

> The Freudian analysts emphasized that their theories were constantly verified by their clinical observations. As for Adler, I was much impressed by a personal experience. Once in 1919, I reported to him a case which to me did not seem particularly Adlerian, but which he found no difficulty in analysing in terms of his theory of inferiority feelings, although he had not even seen the child. Slightly shocked, I asked him how he could be so sure. Because of my thousandfold experience, he replied; whereupon I could not help saying: 'And with this new case, I suppose, your experience has become thousand-and-one-fold' [7].

Popper claims that 'the criterion of the scientific status of a theory is its falsifiability, or refutability, or testability', and psychoanalytical theories do not fulfil this criterion. According to Popper, they constitute a pseudo-science and a collection of myths which contain 'most interesting psychological suggestions, but not in a testable form'; he only offers the consolation 'that historically speaking all—or very nearly all—scientific theories originate from myths, and that a myth may contain important anticipations of scientific theories'. Popper's criticism is particularly harsh and his criterion of falsifiability is problematic, but there can be no doubt that psychoanalysis cannot claim the same scientific status as most theories in somatic medicine.

Psychoanalysis as a hermeneutic discipline

The emphasis in psychoanalysis on the importance of the state of anxiety implies, in agreement with the philosophy of Kierkegaard and Heidegger, that anxiety is an essential feature of the human personality, and that uncritical removal of this symptom, for instance by means of an anxiolytic drug, may constitute a violation of the patient as a person, as it deprives him of the possibility of resolving the neurotic conflict. Since the early 1960s, this connection between psychoanalysis and hermeneutic philosophy has attracted the interest of continental philosophers (e.g. Paul Ricoeur and Jürgen Habermas) and psychoanalysts (e.g. Carl Lesche and Alfred Lorenzer) who oppose the naturalistic point of view and conclude that psychoanalysis must be regarded as a hermeneutic discipline [8–11]. The object of the psychoanalytical enquiry is not the 'hydraulics of the mind', but associations of meanings formulated in language, and the method of psychoanalysis is not the scientific experiment, but understanding, interpretation and reflection.

In order to explain this idea it is necessary to realize that the word 'understanding' has several meanings, and, first, we shall consider the mental operation, which is sometimes called 'empathic understanding'. Imagine that one day you see a person walking down the street. He stops, puts a pipe in his mouth, searches his pockets, crosses the street, enters a tobacconist's shop, comes out with a tin of tobacco in his hand, lights his pipe and proceeds down the street. Anybody will be able to understand the behaviour of this man. He felt 'tobacco hunger', wanted to smoke and, since he had no tobacco, he decided to buy some from the tobacconist's across the road. The interpreter, who arrives at this conclusion, has *internalized* the person's behaviour by putting himself in that person's place, and in this way he has been able to link the sequence of events in a rational way. Even an interpreter who is a non-smoker will be able to understand the smoker's behaviour: he will have experienced other types of 'hunger' and he will recognize the *behaviour maxim* that those who feel hunger try to allay that feeling by appropriate action. Theodore Abel, who discusses a similar case, concludes:

> By specifying the steps which are implicit in the interpretation of our case, we have brought out two particulars which are characteristic of the act of *Verstehen* [understanding]. One is the 'internalizing' of observed factors in a given situation; the other is the application of a behaviour maxim which makes the connection between these factors relevant. Thus we 'understand' a given human action if we can apply to it a generalization based upon personal experience [12].

The crucial problem is, of course, that it is impossible to prove with absolute certainty that even the most simple interpretation is correct. One may ask other bystanders what they thought of the pipe smoker's behaviour and, if they arrived at the same conclusion, the interpretation has at least attained the status of an 'inter-subjective truth', but it cannot be excluded that all the observers were wrong. The ultimate test is to ask the pipe smoker himself why he acted as he did, and, if he confirms the interpretation, we may feel almost certain that we were right. It is, however, still possible that the pipe smoker did not speak the truth, but slipped into the shop in order to avoid an unpleasant encounter in the street. Nevertheless, empathic understanding is an indispensable component of communication between human beings in everyday life, and it also plays an important role when doctors communicate with their patients.

This example suggests that to understand simply means 'to imagine oneself in somebody else's shoes' and 'to share the feelings of that person', but, as we have explained in detail in the preceding chapter, hermeneutic philosophers do not stop here. An analytical hermeneuticist, like Peter Winch, regards understanding as knowledge. The sociologist who is visiting the Trobriand Islands may describe the daily activities of the islanders, but empathic understanding based on personal experience is not sufficient to make him interpret what goes on; understanding presupposes a thorough knowledge of the language and rules of behaviour of that particular culture which differs markedly from his own. Heidegger's and Gadamer's point of view was also explained. For Heidegger, the process of understanding is not just one kind of mental activity among many others, with which one may occupy oneself; understanding and interpretation are constituent features of human nature in the sense that the very concept of conscious awareness implies that we are engaged in understanding and interpreting the world in which we find ourselves (Chapter 9). A conscious human being by necessity establishes a horizon of understanding, and, according to Gadamer, two people only fully understand each other, if their horizons of understanding have fused.

These ideas are important to all those psychiatrists who do not content themselves with studying the behaviour of their patients and recording the effect of drug treatment on that behaviour, but they cannot be directly applied in all psychiatric cases. The problems of the severely emaciated patient with anorexia nervosa who still refuses to eat, the patient who feels compelled to wash his hands several hundred times each day, and the one who claims that his thoughts are being read by other people, cannot be solved 'by putting oneself in their shoes', by learning their language and form of life, or by seeking a fusion of the psychiatrist's and the patients' horizons of understanding. The psychiatrist cannot directly understand the behaviour of his neurotic and psychotic patients, but needs a key to see the logic and meaning behind the symptoms, and it has been claimed by, among others, the German psychoanalyst Alfred Lorenzer that psychoanalytical theory provides that key [10]. He claims that psychoanalysis is a critical theory about the formation of the personality of the individual, which serves to reconstruct the life history of the patient. Psychoanalysis is concerned with meanings formulated in language and, consequently, it belongs to the humanities rather than to the natural sciences. Lorenzer also stresses that the purpose of psychoanalysis is not only to free the patients from their disabling symptoms, but also to increase their self-understanding and social competence and to promote a critical attitude towards those conditions in society which contribute to the development of mental disease. Psychoanalvsis, from Lorenzer's point of view, is a critical theory of the socialization of the individual, and his views are clearly related to those of Habermas (Chapter 10).

The Swedish psychiatrist, Carl Lesche, has described in greater detail in which way psychoanalysis contributes to the hermeneutic process [11], and we shall briefly explain his ideas. A psychoanalytical inquiry, which seeks to explore the unconscious mind, is always impeded by gaps in both co-understanding and self-understanding, and, according to Lesche, psychoanalytical theory serves to bridge those gaps by means of *quasi-naturalistic explanations*. For instance, analysts may say that a certain behaviour is caused by the repression or sublimation of instincts, and in that way they explain otherwise incomprehensible behaviour in a manner which at least superficially resembles causal explanations in natural science. Such explanations, however, deserve the prefix 'quasi', as they do not, like scientific explanations, represent the aim of the inquiry, but serve to mediate understanding. They are subordinated to the hermeneutic interests.

Lesche describes the psychoanalytical process in terms of alternating hermeneutic and quasi-naturalistic phases. At the beginning of the dialogue the analyst and the patient directly understand one another, as they speak the same language and at least to some extent share the same cultural background, and, on the basis of such *pre-understanding*, an attempt is made to map in broad outline the life history of the patient. The reasons for some important decisions in the patient's life will be easily comprehensible, and it will be possible to illuminate important aspects of the patient's personality. Sooner or later, however, a crisis in co-understanding sets in. The analyst, who can no longer see the point of the patient's behaviour or grasp his motives, engages himself in quasi-naturalistic reasoning; he regards the patient's behaviour as a 'natural phenomenon', the causes of which must be explained. For instance, a psychoanalyst who analyses a patient with a phobia, like the woman who dared not touch objects made of rubber, may suspect that this seemingly irrational behaviour is 'caused' by an unconscious conflict between a primitive instinct and the superego, and he will use his skills to steer the dialogue in a manner which is suited to test this hypothesis. If in the end the patient accepts the suggested causes as his or her hidden reasons, the hypothesis has been confirmed as a subjective truth, and the quasi-naturalistic phase has come to an end. Then, communication on the hermeneutic level is resumed until the next crisis sets in.

According to this view, the id and the superego are not entities which are given empirically, and repression is not due to some kind of mechanical force, but these and other psychoanalytical concepts are those categories within which the analyst reasons when he tries to interpret the dynamics of the patient's personality. To use Lorenzer's and Lesche's terminology, the psychoanalytical concepts constitute a *meta-hermeneutic* language (*meta* = behind, beyond), i.e. the language which provides the key to the hermeneutic process. The resulting interpretations are true, if the patient recognizes them as the truth, and they evade objective proof.

A balanced view

It is very difficult to define in exact terms the philosophical status of psychoanalytical theories, but an analysis of the arguments of the critics may help us to formulate a balanced view.

The empiricist philosophers who belonged to the Vienna circle were much concerned with the formulation of a *demarcation criterion* in order to distinguish between those statements which are meaningful and those which are not, and, as explained in Chapter 2, they chose the criterion of verifiability. Obviously, it is impossible to imagine any observation which can verify the objective truth of a psychoanalytical interpretation, and, therefore, psychoanalysis must, from the empiricist point of view, be deemed meaningless. Analysts like Freud and Adler (p. 161), of course, would not have accepted this conclusion, as they asserted that their theories were constantly verified by their clinical observations, but the true empiricist would object to the analysts' use of the word observation, as the analysts were not referring to sense experience, but to their subjective interpretation of their patients' answers and reactions during the analysis. We agree that psychoanalytical theories and interpretations cannot be verified by means of our senses, but we reject the empiricists' assertion that non-verifiable statements are never meaningful. Statements about motives, intentions, wishes and values are not verifiable by observation, but they are not necessarily devoid of meaning.

Popper also chose a demarcation criterion, but there are two differences between his line of reasoning and that of the empiricists. Firstly, Popper chose the criterion of falsifiability and we have already discussed the logical implications of the distinction between falsification and verification (p. 22). In this particular context, however, the distinction is relatively unimportant, as psychoanalytical statements can neither be verified nor falsified by observation. Secondly, Popper does not use his demarcation criterion to distinguish between those statements which are meaningful and those which are not, but to separate scientific from non-scientific statements, and that is an important point. We fully agree with Popper in so far as he concludes that psychoanalysis is non-scientific, i.e. that it does not belong to the natural sciences, but his criticism goes further than that. He does not just state that psychoanalytical theory is non-scientific, though perhaps meaningful; he asserts that it is a collection of myths, and that claim is more doubtful. If he simply means that *contemporary* psychoanalytical theories are no more than a collection of myths, we shall not object too strongly; the number of theories is vast, they are to a large extent incompatible, and at present it seems impossible to separate the wheat from the chaff. If, however, Popper is implying that, in the nature of things, psychoanalytical theory must always remain a collection of myths, we disagree. The psychoanalyst tries to explore those connections of meanings, which may explain the patient's symptoms, and the contention that such an endeavour is doomed to failure seems unwarranted.

There are several reasons for our critical attitude to contemporary psychoanalysis, and we shall discuss some of these.

Sometimes, psychoanalytical theories seem to be formulated in such a way that they are logically non-refutable, and, as pointed out by Germund Hesslow, Freud's theory of dreams is a possible example [13]. According to that theory, all dreams represent wish-fulfilments (or attempted wish-fulfilments), which means that we dream what we wish, even though we may not dare admit to ourselves in the waking state that we have such wishes. This is a rather attractive theory as it suggests that dreaming is always pleasant, but unfortunately most of us also remember highly unpleasant dreams—nightmares—which made us wake up in a sweat. The disinterested critic would be tempted to conclude that such experiences represent a refutation of the hypothesis that dreams are wish-fulfilments, but Freudian psychoanalysts to some extent 'immunize' their theory by claiming that unpleasant dreams may reflect our masochistic dispositions. Of course, it is logically possible that everybody has such dispositions, but as yet the hypothesis has not been 'tested' by studies of a large number of individuals in whom the occurrence of unpleasant dreams was correlated with other signs of masochistic tendencies. Psychoanalytical theories cannot be verified or falsified experimentally, but it is a minimum requirement that their internal coherence is ascertained by studies of groups of people.

It also presents a problem that psychoanalysts tend to validate their theories by the publication of a few case histories. Freud, for instance, illustrates his paranoia theory by the case of Schreber [14], and his hysteria theory by the cases of Anna O., Elisabeth von R. and Dora. The validity of such generalizations from individual cases seems very doubtful, as it is hard to believe that psychiatric symptoms (e.g. paranoia) do not have as many 'causes' as somatic symptoms (e.g. chest pain). Once again, it may be claimed that systematic studies of groups of patients are needed to examine as critically as possible the justification of the theories. According to the paranoia theory, for instance, the psychiatric symptoms are 'caused' by suppressed homosexual tendencies, and studies which compare the occurrence of overt homosexuality in patients suffering from paranoia and patients suffering from other mental diseases might yield interesting results. Psychoanalysts, however, do not seem to reason in this way. They often argue that all their patients are different and that the truth of their interpretations emerges from the reaction of the individual patient during the analysis, but that does not prevent them from writing books in which they generalize their ideas.

Usually, psychoanalysts also reject all attempts to test the effect of psychoanalysis empirically, but it must be remembered that analysts do not only claim that their patients learn to understand themselves, but also that they are relieved of their phobias and other symptoms and that their social competence is enhanced. In

Psychoanalysis: Natural Science or Hermeneutics? 169

other words, it is claimed that the patients' behaviour is changed, and that claim invites empirical testing by means of randomized controlled trials in order to compare the efficacy of psychoanalysis, other forms of psychotherapy and perhaps drug treatment. Evidence of this kind is scarce, but many uncontrolled series of treatment results have been published. In 1965, Eysenck reviewed nineteen studies of the efficiency of individual psychotherapy, including both classical psychoanalysis and a number of eclectic versions, and he concluded that these studies, which in all comprised more than 7000 patients, did not support the assertion that it is possible to cure neurotic patients by means of such methods [15]. In 1980, Rachman and Wilson reviewed the literature once again and their conclusion is almost as negative. They state that 'modest evidence now supports the claim that psychotherapy is capable of producing some beneficial changes—but the negative results still outnumber the positive findings, and both of these are exceeded by reports that are beyond interpretation' [16].

We are not implying by these points of criticism that psychoanalysis in principle must be rejected, but only that an effort must be made to change the present state of affairs.

First of all, agreement must be reached as regards the theoretical status of psychoanalytical theory, and at present Lorenzer's and Lesche's approach seems the most promising. They stress correctly that psychoanalysis is a hermeneutic discipline, and they provide a plausible explanation of the role of psychoanalytical theory: it is, to use Lorenzer's expression, the meta-language which is required to guide the hermeneutic process. It is to be hoped that further development of psychoanalytical theory along these lines may help psychiatrists to communicate with their patients even under those circumstances when empathic understanding fails. Psychiatrists see patients with a variety of symptoms (e.g. hysterical paralyses, delusions, obsessions, compulsions and unexplained anxiety) and psychoanalysis may enable them to see the mental state of the individual patient as the result of a dynamic process; psychoanalysis may permit an interpretation of seemingly bizarre symptoms in the context of the patient's past and present history, i.e. the development of the patient's personality during childhood and adolescence, the patient's interaction with others in later life, and the influence of recent social events. Lorenzer and Lesche are clearly right when they stress that psychiatrists must concern themselves with meanings formulated in language, and when they reject the attempts of biologically orientated psychiatrists and behaviourists to reduce all mental disease to abnormal brain function and inappropriate behaviour.

In the last chapter of this book we shall discuss a mind–body theory which is called *functionalism*, and that theory may also illuminate the status of psychoanalysis. As we shall explain, functionalists compare the relationship between mental states and the physiological states of the brain with that between a computer program and the computer 'hardware', and the mental processes of the neurotic or psychotic mind may well be regarded as the product of an 'abnormal computer program'. If that analogy is accepted, the concepts of psychoanalytical theory (e.g. ego, superego, repression and projection) may be said to represent those concepts which are needed to 'decipher' the programs of the patients' minds.

Psychoanalysts must also learn to accept that empirical proof is needed when they claim that their methods have observable beneficial effects, and they must learn from natural scientists to adopt a more critical attitude to their theories [17]. The indisputable fact that the truth of a psychoanalytic theory is subjective rather than objective, must not be regarded as a *carte blanche* to extravagant speculation.

Notes and References

1 Cameron, N. *Personality Development and Psychopathology*. Boston: Houghton Mifflin, 1963.
2 Quoted from Hall, C.S. *A Primer of Freudian Psychology*. New York: New American Library, 1954, pp. 65–6.
3 Jaspers, K. *General Psychopathology*. Manchester: Manchester University Press, 1972, p. 774.
4 Hartmann, H. *Essay on Ego Psychology*. New York: International University Press, 1964.
5 Freud, S. *Introductory Lectures on Psychoanalysis* (Standard edition, Vol. XV). London: Hogarth Press, 1981, p. 193.
6 Quoted from Luborsky, L. & Spence, D.P. Quantitative research on psychoanalytic therapy. In: Garfield, S.L. & Bergin, A.E. (eds) *Handbook of Psychotherapy and Behavior Change*. New York: Wiley, 1978, pp. 356–7.
7 Popper, K.R. *Conjectures and Refutations*, 2nd edn. London: Routledge and Kegan Paul, 1965, pp. 35–8.

8   Ricoeur, P. *De l'interprétation*. Paris: Editions du Seul, 1965.
9   Habermas, J. *Knowledge and Human Interests*. London: Heinemann, 1972.
10 Lorenzer, A. *Die Wahrheit der psychoanalytischen Erkenntnis*. Frankfurt am Main: Suhrkamp, 1976.
11 Lesche, C. Some metascientific reflections on the difference between psychoanalysis and psychotherapy. *Scandinavian Psychoanalytical Review*, 1978; 1: 147–81.
12 Abel, T. The operation called 'Verstehen'. *American Journal of Sociology*, 1948–9; 54: 211–8.
13 Hesslow, G. *Medicinsk Vetenskapsteori*. Lund: Studentlitteratur, 1979, pp. 141–3.
14 Freud, S. *Psycho-Analytic Notes on an Autobiographical Account of a Case of Paranoia (Dementia Paranoides)* (Standard edition, Vol. XII). London: Hogarth Press, 1981, pp. 9–82.
15 Eysenck, H.J. The effects of psychotherapy. *International Journal of Psychiatry*, 1965; 1: 97–178.
16 Rachman, S.J. & Wilson, G.T. *The Effects of Psychological Therapy*, 2nd edn. Oxford: Pergamon, 1980, pp. 259.
17 Some doctors, especially general practitioners, medical sociologists and psychiatrists, stress the need for qualitative research, as opposed to traditional quantitative research. Unfortunately, the concept of qualitative research is extremely ill-defined, but, among other things, it includes semi-structured interview studies in which the interviewer takes an interest in the attitudes, feelings and motives of the interviewed persons. It might be more fruitful to distinguish between this type of research, which may well be labelled 'hermeneutic' and the traditional 'scientific' kind of medical research.

CHAPTER 12
MEDICAL ETHICS AS A PHILOSOPHICAL DISCIPLINE

For a period of three months, the doctors from the medical unit at a large Danish hospital made a note each time they encountered what was called a *significant ethical problem* [1]. A problem was regarded as ethical if it involved a non-technical value judgment, and it was labelled significant if the clinician felt in doubt about which decision to make, or if he or she believed that other clinicians might have evaluated the problem differently. During those three months, 426 patients were admitted to the unit and in 25% of those cases the doctors felt that they were confronted with one or more significant ethical problems. The clinicians were often in doubt whether or not it was warranted to reduce the usual diagnostic or therapeutic activity in old or chronically ill patients, whose future quality of life was judged to be poor, and they often found it difficult to decide what to tell patients with a newly diagnosed malignant disease.

However, the spectrum of ethical dilemmas was vast and included questions like these: what does one do when a patient needs surgical treatment in order to save her life, but refuses blood transfusions for religious reasons, or when a patient wants to go on driving his car when he is not considered fit to do so? What is the right decision when a patient, who is quite unable to take care of herself, refuses to be transferred to a nursing home, and what does a doctor tell a patient who has been treated incorrectly by a colleague and wants to hear the doctor's opinion about that treatment? This survey clearly showed that everyday clinical decision-making has an important ethical dimension. Clinicians are not only concerned with scientific problems, like making a diagnosis or choosing the most effective treatment.

Medical ethics belongs to the borderland between medicine and philosophy, and it constitutes one of those areas where cooperation between doctors and philosophers may prove most fruitful. It is a medical discipline in so far as the problems to be solved are medical ones, but it is also a philosophical discipline as many of the problems are just special cases of ethical quandaries which have been discussed by moral philosophers for centuries. In this chapter we shall approach the topic from a philosophical angle, and in the following one we shall apply some of the philosophical concepts and ideas to medical problems.

'Good' and 'ought'

The clinician who is faced with an ethical dilemma must decide what he *ought* to do and which action is *best* for the patient. Words like 'good' and 'ought'—and their derivatives—are keywords in all ethical analyses, and in order to explain their meaning in moral contexts we shall for the moment discuss the game of chess [2]. This game may be regarded as a social institution with a code of its own, comprising a set of values and a set of rules. The absolute values which characterize the game are extremely simple as it is good to win, less good to play stalemate and bad to lose. If we regard this institution from the outside, we may, of course, ask why it is good to win and bad to lose, but, if we place ourselves inside the institution and think, as a chess player does, it makes no sense to ask the question. It simply is a constituent feature of the game that it is good to win; it is, in the terminology of moral philosophy, *good in itself*. However, the word 'good' may also be used in a different sense. During the game, the chess player may tell us that some moves are good and that others are bad for developing a certain strategy, but here the word is used in a relative or technical sense. The good move is not good in itself, but *good as a means,* as it cannot be excluded that the strategy fails and that the end-result of the game is not good at all.

It is also part of the game that a chess player ought only to move the bishop diagonally and, when we are thinking within the institution, as a chess player does, it again makes no sense to ask why this is so. It is a constituent feature of the game that bishops must be moved in that particular manner; it is, to apply Kant's terminology to the microcosm of the chess board, *a categorical imperative* [3]. However, a chess player may also decide that he ought to move an unprotected pawn which is being attacked, but that is a different kind of ought. It means that he ought to move the chess piece *if* he does not want to lose it, and, consequently, it is not a categorical but a *hypothetical imperative*. It is not against the rules to lose a pawn and it may even be part of the player's strategy to sacrifice that piece in order to win the game.

Of course, we do not wish to imply that life in general is like a chess game with fixed rules and values, but the example illustrates, albeit crudely, that words like 'good' and 'ought' (as well as similar expressions like better, worse, right and wrong) are sometimes used in their ethical sense (the ultimate good and the categorical ought) and sometimes in their non-ethical sense.

In medicine we may say that an antibiotic is good or effective for killing certain bacteria, and in that context good signifies *good as a means*. However, doctors sometimes wonder if it would not be *better* in some cases to withhold effective therapy; the future prospects for the patient may be so poor that it is considered *best* for the patient to die from an intercurrent infection. Here the words 'better' and 'best' have their full ethical meaning, as the doctor is considering the ultimate values in the human chess game.

The different meanings of the word 'ought' are well illustrated by the statement, 'The obstetrician ought not to do an abortion'. The person who made this statement might mean that it is morally forbidden to do an abortion and in that case it is meant as a categorical imperative, but the statement may also mean that the obstetrician ought not to do the abortion *if* he does not want to break the law, or *if* he does not wish to expose the patient to a particular complication. If one of these interpretations is the correct one, the ought-sentence was only meant as a hypothetical imperative. The example shows that the norms which govern our actions need not be *moral*, but that they may be *legal* or *technical*. Confusion arises when this distinction is forgotten.

Ethics on three levels

The discussion so far served to show what ethics is all about, but we have already left far too many questions unanswered, and it will be necessary to proceed more systematically. Traditionally, philosophers distinguish between *descriptive ethics, meta-ethics* and *normative ethics* and, although this distinction is by no means sharp, it helps to systematize the presentation.

The survey which was quoted at the beginning of this chapter illustrates what is understood by descriptive ethics. We counted and classified those ethical problems which clinicians face in their daily routine, and we might also have recorded which decisions the clinicians actually made in different situations. Such studies differ little from other empirical studies which serve to describe the world as it is.

Meta-ethics, on the other hand, is a purely philosophical discipline which concerns the meaning and logical status of ethical concepts and arguments. Those who engage themselves in meta-ethical investigations may discuss to what extent moral values are part of the fabric of the world and to what extent they must be regarded as conventions, emotions or prescriptions, but they do not specify which things are good and what is the right action in a particular situation.

Normative ethics is also a philosophical discipline, but it concerns our *actual moral attitudes* and deals with the formulation and justification of moral principles. Thus, moral philosophers who concern themselves with normative ethics may tell us which duties we must accept in our daily lives and what in their opinion is morally good. As we shall see later, there are several mutually conflicting normative systems. Some philosophers tell us only to stress the consequences of our actions (utilitarian ethics), whereas others claim that some principles, e.g. justice and certain duties and rights, are morally compelling regardless of the consequences (deontological ethics). Many ethical problems in medicine represent conflicts between utilitarian and deontological considerations, and it is one of the most difficult problems in moral philosophy to decide whether utilitarian and deontological ethics can be reconciled.

The origin of morality

In this presentation we shall adopt the meta-ethical assumption that moral values, principles and codes are human constructions which are built into our social and legal institutions, and serve to regulate our dealings with one another.

The British philosopher, J. L. Mackie, states that the human predicament is such that things are liable to go badly:

> ... badly in the natural non-moral sense that human wants, needs and interests are likely to be frustrated in large measure.
> ... Men sometimes display active malevolence to one another, but even apart from that they are almost always more concerned with their selfish ends than with helping one another. The function of morality is primarily to counteract this limitation of man's sympathy [4].

Human beings forming a society must by necessity create a moral code which, with minor or major changes, is transmitted from generation to generation. Early in life we have been taught a set of values and a set of duties, and such norms may be incorporated into our way of thinking to such an extent that we are led to the false belief that they represent eternal truths.

This view of the origin of morality need not imply that moral norms are purely subjective. Moral values and principles may not be part of the fabric of the world in the same way as mountains and trees, but they may still be regarded as objective in the sense that they constitute a social reality. Similarly, moral statements may not be true or false in the same way as statements about the weight and length of a physical object, but they may be subjected to rational discussion and, by the application of the rules of logic, it may be found that they are consistent or inconsistent with some generally accepted moral principle.

It follows from this argument that it would be wrong to adopt the relativistic point of view that one moral code is as acceptable as any other. Moral codes or systems have numerous components and their moral validity depends on the degree of internal coherence, i.e. to which extent the components are mutually consistent. It is required, for instance, that our actual moral attitudes are consistent with our meta-ethical assumptions and, therefore, the medical ethicist must concern himself with both normative ethics and meta-ethics.

An acceptable set of moral principles must also take into account empirical facts. A code of medical ethics, for instance, must reflect among other things, the organization of the health service, the level of education of the population, and, not to forget, the state of medical knowledge and technology. The moral code which was developed by doctors in Ancient Greece does not provide sufficient guidance to 20th century doctors, and even today medical ethics must of necessity change gradually, as new technological advances create new ethical problems.

Some doctors will disagree strongly with our meta-ethical assumption that morality is a human construction which is at the same time a social reality, and we shall briefly present other meta-ethical positions, which have had considerable influence on medical thinking. The doctor who accepts the *traditional Christian view* will object to the assertion that moral rules are human constructions. Bliss and Johnson describe the belief of the Christian with these words:

> He believes that there must be an external standard of reference and that those moral principles have been revealed by God in the form of commandments, but, more than that, he believes that the principles have been clearly demonstrated in the life and teaching of Jesus Christ [5].

According to this position, the moral code is something to be discovered, whereas according to our view it is something to be made.

Immanuel Kant (1724-1804) is one of those philosophers who have asserted most strongly that man is the legislator of morality, and the following quotation from the *Foundation of the Metaphysics of Morals* illustrates well the difference between that position and the traditional Christian one:

> If we look back upon all previous attempts which have ever been undertaken to discover the principle of morality, it is not to be wondered at all that they have all had to fail. Man was seen to be bound by laws to his duty, but it was not seen that he is subject only to his own, yet universal, legislation, and that he is only bound to act in accordance with his own will, which is, however, designed by nature to be a will giving universal laws [6].

It will be noticed that the presentation of medical ethics in this book is strongly influenced by Kant's view.

At the other extreme, there are the *emotivists* who reject all attempts to reason about ethical problems, as they believe that moral statements express no more than the personal taste of the speaker. Bertrand Russell writes:

> This doctrine consists in maintaining that, if two men differ about values there is not a disagreement as to any kind of truth, but a difference of taste. If one man says 'oysters are good' and another says 'oysters are bad', we recognize that there is nothing to argue about. The theory in question holds that all differences as to values are of this sort, although we naturally do not think so when we are dealing with matters that seem to us more exalted than oysters [7].

Emotivism is linked to the empiricist point of view that only those statements are meaningful which can be tested by experience: the truth of moral statements is not testable and therefore they are devoid of meaning. Few philosophers today will accept this reasoning, but empiricism—in the form of logical positivism—has been very influential in medicine, and that may explain why scientifically minded doctors for many years have paid little attention to the analysis of the ethical dimension of medical problems.

Finally, there are the *ethical naturalists* who—in contrast to the adherents of all the other schools of thought—deny the distinction between value judgments and empirical facts, as they believe that words like 'good' and 'ought' can be reduced to empirical features of the natural world, such as happiness or human desires. Naturalistic meta-ethics is closely linked to utilitarian normative ethics, which we shall discuss later, and, in the last century, Jeremy Bentham went so far as to suggest that it might be possible to calculate which decision in a particular situation produces the greatest amount of happiness. It is interesting that contemporary medical decision theorists think along exactly the same lines, as they believe that it is sometimes possible to calculate which is the best medical decision by means of sophisticated utility theory and cost-benefit analyses [8].

The mechanical model of disease, according to which value-laden concepts like illness and health are reduced to biological phenomena (Chapter 4), is yet another version of naturalism in medicine.

The structure of ethical reasoning

Theories of normative ethics fall into two main groups: *consequentialist* (or *utilitarian*) theories and *deontological* theories (from Greek *deon* = duty), and we shall discuss some of these, partly by means of non-medical examples.

Consider the following cases:

1. I am trying to make up my mind how to vote at a general election. In the end I decide to vote for one particular political party, as I believe that it will be best for the greatest possible number of people in my country, if that party is strengthened.
2. In a particular situation I am trying to make up my mind whether I should tell the truth or tell a lie. I decide that withholding the truth will have the best consequences, and I tell a lie.

In both situations the decision-maker *chooses that action which in his opinion has the best consequences for the greatest possible number of people,* and this way of reasoning, which probably is familiar to everybody, is called *universal act utilitarianism*. We shall briefly explain these words. It is an example of *utilitarian* thinking, as the decision-maker only takes into account the consequences or the utility of his action and ignores all other considerations. He does not, for instance, consider the possibility that it might be his duty to tell the truth, regardless of the consequences. Further, the strategy is called *act* utilitarian, as the decision-maker only considers the consequences of this particular act, and it is labelled *universal* as he considers the consequences for everybody concerned and not for any particular person or persons. That version of utilitarianism was originally proposed by Jeremy Bentham (1748–1832) and, as explained above, it is closely linked to meta-ethical naturalism, as it is assumed that moral values can be reduced to the feeling of happiness. Later utilitarian philosophers, like John Stuart Mill (1808–73), have rejected the simplistic idea that happiness is the goal of all human activity and have argued that there are other values as well, such as the freedom of the individual, truth, health, aesthetic experience and friendship. This necessary refinement of utilitarian thinking immediately creates the difficulty that we are then forced to compare different kinds of goodness. We shall see later that this is one of the main problems of utilitarian thinking in medicine.

Other utilitarian philosophers have argued that it is simply not possible to predict the consequences of a particular action and that it is an essential feature of moral behaviour to base one's decisions on action principles or moral *rules*. To illustrate this idea we may elaborate on the previous example:

> I am wondering whether I should tell the truth or a lie, and I still believe that telling a lie in this case would have the best consequences. However, I also believe that the consequences would be very bad, if everybody started telling lies, and, therefore, my final decision is to tell the truth.

This strategy, which is called *universal rule utilitarianism,* was suggested by the philosopher of law, John Austin (1790–1859). The decision-maker no longer asks, 'What are the likely consequences of my action in this particular situation?', but he reasons in a more roundabout way, 'What principles are involved in my decision, and what would the general consequences be, if everybody acted according to those principles?' We shall show in the next chapter that this strategy is important when doctors wish to consider the wider consequences of their actions [9].

Consequentialist thinking may, however, also take other forms, as it is not self-evident that one must always consider the general consequences of one's action and not just the consequences for oneself or somebody else. In the case of the general election one might, for instance, argue like this:

> I am trying to make up my mind how to vote at a general election, and in the end I decide to vote for one particular party, as I believe that it will serve my interests best.

This strategy deserves the name *ethical egoism,* and the immediate impression may well be that it represents the opposite of moral behaviour. However, much contemporary political philosophy is based on the idea that everybody has the right to pursue his own happiness, as long as he permits others to do the same, and with that important constraint egoism must not necessarily be condemned.

The final example of consequentialist thinking is perhaps the most important from a medical point of view:

> I have the choice between giving my patient treatment A and treatment B, and I decide to give him treatment A as I believe

that it will have the best consequences for him.

This strategy may be called *patient-orientated utilitarianism*, as the doctor, in accordance with his professional duty, restricts his considerations to the consequences for his patient. It is seen that in the case of both ethical egoism and patient-orientated utilitarianism, the restriction of the considerations to one person is connected with the acknowledgment of certain rights and duties, which means that it is bound up with deontological considerations.

The *deontologist* tells us that the assessment of the consequences of our actions does not constitute the supreme moral principle as other considerations take priority. For instance, we read in the Old Testament that 'thou shalt not bear false witness against thy neighbour', and, if we accept this divine commandment, it is beside the point to discuss the consequences of telling a lie; it is simply our duty to tell the truth, regardless of the consequences.

In modern philosophy the deontological point of view can be traced to Kant. In Kant's philosophy morality is firmly based on the concept of man as a rational being with a free will, and the supreme moral principle is not the assessment of the consequences of our actions, but the respect for the persons involved. We explained in the introduction to this chapter that in chess it is a 'categorical imperative' to move the bishop diagonally on the chess board, and, according to Kant, there is only one categorical imperative when human beings deal with one another. In one of Kant's phrases 'Act so that you treat humanity, whether in your own person or in that of another, always as an end and never as a means only' [10].

A rational being exists as an end in itself, and using a person as a means is the same as violating his humanity and treating him as a thing. This concept of man, which resembles Kierkegaard's concept (Chapter 9), has gained wide acceptance in medical ethics, and it follows from this idea that maximization of the utility of our actions must be regarded as unethical, if the dignity, integrity or rights of the person involved are violated. Utilitarian assessments are subordinate to Kant's categorical imperative.

Kant also formulates the categorical imperative in a different way, which may be paraphrased as follows: 'I should never act in such a way that I could not will that my maxim should be a universal law', which implies, among other things, that we must treat others as we expect them to treat us [11].

This wording reveals particularly well the duality of Kantian ethics: it is *individualistic* (as man 'is only bound according to his own will'), but at the same time it is based on universal *rules* (as those 'laws' which are deduced from the categorical imperative are universally valid). Kant argues, for instance, that the telling of lies is immoral, and that each of us must arrive at that conclusion when we apply the categorical imperative.

We shall now briefly introduce two deontological theories which are very different, but are both inspired by Kant. The contemporary American philosopher, John Rawls, is not so much concerned with individual action as with the organization of society, and his theory is an attempt to deal with the problem, which was discussed on page 176, that 'the human predicament is such that things are liable to go badly' and that human beings living together need a moral code to regulate their self-interests. Rawls seeks a supreme moral principle which is acceptable to rational, self-interested people and arrives at the conclusion that the fundamental moral notion is that of *social justice* or *fairness*. In the introduction to his monumental book *A Theory of Justice* he writes:

> Justice is the first virtue of social institutions, as truth is of systems of thought. A theory however elegant and economical must be rejected or revised if it is untrue; likewise laws and institutions no matter how efficient and well-arranged must be reformed or abolished if they are unjust. Each person possesses an inviolability founded on justice that even the welfare of society as a whole cannot override [12].

Rawls suggests that the justice or fairness of social practices may be tested by means of a thought experiment. We are asked to imagine a group of persons who come together to establish the practices and organization of a society of which they are to become members, and that their discussions take place 'under a veil of ignorance'. This means that they must commit themselves in a hypothetical state of ignorance about, for instance, the place in society they are going to occupy, their own fortune in the distribution of natural assets and abilities, and their psychological features such as an aversion to risk or liability to optimism and pessimism [13].

Those principles which are acceptable to such people, who are trying to safeguard their own interests under the veil of ignorance, must be regarded as fair and may be incorporated into a *social contract*, which it is the duty of all members of society to obey. Thus, Rawls's version of rule deontology is a social contract theory. He further argues that the resulting contract must be based on the following two important principles:

1 Each person is to have an equal right to the most extensive liberty compatible with a similar liberty for others [14].
2 Social and economic inequalities are to be arranged so that they are ... to the greatest benefit of the least advantaged ... [15].

These principles express justice as a complex of three ideas: liberty, equality, and reward for contributions to the common advantage [16].

Rawls himself asserts that his ideas are compatible with those of Kant [17, 18] and, like Kant, he is opposed to utilitarian thinking. As an example, he discusses slavery, which may be defended on utilitarian grounds if the advantages to the slaveholders outweigh the disadvantages to the slaves, whereas his second principle, in accordance with our moral intuitions, forbids this practice as the inequalities in the slave state are not to the greatest benefit of the least advantaged. In the next chapter we shall apply Rawls's ideas when we discuss the general principles of medical ethics and the moral basis of the organization of health services, whereas the individualistic aspect of Kant's deontology is particularly important when we discuss the management of the individual patient.

Both Kant and Rawls may be called rule deontologists, as they believe that it is possible to formulate general moral principles, and, to complete the picture, we shall briefly mention a radically different position, Sartre's act deontology.

Jean-Paul Sartre (1905–80) agrees with Kant that 'man is only bound to act according to his own will', but he takes this thesis so seriously that he denies the existence of universal laws which can be applied at the moment of decision. He claims that 'man creates himself; he is not complete from the beginning, he creates himself by choosing his own morality' [19].

In his book *Existentialism and Humanism* Sartre relates that once during the Second World War one of his pupils asked for his advice. The pupil had the choice between staying with his mother, who needed help, and leaving for England to join the Free French Forces. If he left, his mother would die, and, if he stayed, he would have failed his country. Sartre replied, 'I have only one answer to give: you are free, choose yourself, that is, think of something! No universal moral can tell you what to do! [20].

The only help which we can offer somebody who has to make a difficult decision is to make clear the actual circumstances which constitute the premises of the choice. The person himself must make the choice and bear the consequences.

This radical theory, which questions the possibility of ethical reasoning, will be unacceptable to most people, but it illustrates well the extreme views of some hermeneutic philosophers.

The wide reflective equilibrium

We have pointed out that a set of moral beliefs must be mutually consistent, that our decisions depend on the moral principles which we accept, and that those principles reflect our meta-ethical assumptions. Thus, no sharp distinction can be made between normative ethics and meta-ethics. Medical ethicists, unlike medical scientists, do not hope to establish the truth, but they seek what Norman Daniels has called *a wide reflective equilibrium* [21]. The aim of their efforts is coherence, and a wide reflective equilibrium may be defined as a coherent system of (a) moral judgments and intuitions in relation to practical experience, (b) moral principles, such as maximization of utility or deontological rules, and (c) background theories about man and society.

All doctors who have seriously tried to analyse the ethical foundation of their decisions will have to admit that it is often difficult to reconcile their intuitions with their various duties, e.g. their duty to choose that decision which has the best consequences for the patient, the duty to respect the patient's autonomy, and, especially if they are working in a national health service with a fixed budget, the duty to ensure that everybody gets a fair deal. However, it is not even sufficient that all members of the medical profession agree on a coherent moral code which covers all these problems, as the code must also be acceptable to their patients. A system of medical ethics cannot be viewed in isolation, but must be harmonized with the general norms and values of that particular society. Doctors sometimes forget this and believe that international codes of ethics express ethical 'truths' which are internationally valid just like scientific truths. On closer inspection, however, it will be found that either such codes are much too vague to offer guidance in clinical practice, or they reflect the moral beliefs in a particular cultural setting, usually Europe and North America.

In spite of all these difficulties, we maintain that it is the ultimate goal of ethical studies to establish a wide reflective equilibrium, just as it is the ultimate goal of science to establish the full truth, but we must also admit that in both cases the goal is unattainable. Ethical problems in medicine are extremely diverse and the development of new technology continually creates new problems, so that it is necessary, again and again, to rethink the system on all levels, in much the same way as the scientist must, again and again, rethink his theories in the light of the results of new experiments.

Therefore, it would be much too much to expect that we should be able, in this chapter and the next one, to present anything like a coherent system of medical ethics, but we have made some assertions which we believe are mutually consistent and which may therefore constitute the rudiments of such a system. We shall conclude this chapter with a brief summary of the most important of those views.

The moral values and norms, which are incorporated into our social institutions and serve to regulate our dealings with one another, are regarded as a human construction. Nevertheless, they are objective in the sense that they constitute a social reality, and they must be justified by rational dialogue.

Medical ethics must be based on Kierkegaard's and Kant's concept of man as a self-reflecting being with a free will, and, consequently, utilitarian considerations must usually give way to those considerations which concern the autonomy of the individual and the justice of social practices. It may be added that we do not exclude the possibility that autonomous people may accept practices which permit others to act on their behalf under certain circumstances.

In the following chapter we shall apply these ideas to medical problems.

Notes and references

1 Kollemorten, I., Strandberg, C., Thomsen, B.M. *et al.* Ethical aspects of clinical decision-making. *Journal of Medical Ethics*, 1981; 7: 67–9.
2 In this book the words *ethical* and *moral* are used as synonyms.
3 This unorthodox example does not do justice to Kant. As we shall explain later, *the* categorical imperative in Kantian ethics is the supreme moral principle. Kant characterizes the categorical imperative as follows: 'Finally, there is one imperative which directly commands a certain conduct without making its condition some purpose to be reached by it. This imperative is categorical.' p. 240 in [6] (p. 416 in the Akademie edition).
4 Mackie, J.L. *Ethics. Inventing Right and Wrong.* Harmondsworth: Penguin Books, 1977, p. 107.
Morality).
5 Bliss, B.P. & Johnson, A.G. *Aims and Motives in Clinical Medicine.* London: Pitman Medical, 1975, p.6.
6 Kant, I. *Grundlegung zur Metaphysik der Sitten* (Originally published 1785). English translation by L. W. Beck. *Foundation of the Metaphysics of Morals.* In: Johnson, O.E. (ed.): *Ethics. Selections from Classical and Contemporary Writers*, 4th edn. New York: Holt, Rinehart & Winston, 1978, p. 246 (p. 432 in the Akademie edition).
7 Russell, B. *Religion and Science.* Oxford: Oxford University Press, 1972.
8 Weinstein, M.C. & Fineberg, H.V. *Clinical Decision Analysis.* Philadelphia: W.B. Saunders, 1980.
9 Some philosophers claim that in principle there is no difference between act and rule utilitarianism (cf. pp. 136–9 in [4]).
10 p. 245 in [6] (p. 429 in the Akademie edition).
11 cf. p. 247 in [6] (p. 434 in the Akademie edition).
12 Rawls, J. *A Theory of Justice.* Oxford: Oxford University Press, 1972, p. 3.
13 p. 137 in [12].
14 p. 60 in [12].
15 p. 83 in [12].
16 Rawls, J. Justice as fairness. *Journal of Philosophy*, 1956; 54: 653–62.
17 p. 251–8 in [12].
18 Rawls, J. Kantian constructivism in moral theory. *Journal of Philosophy*, 1980; 77: 510–72.
19 Sartre, J.-P. *L'existentialisme est un humanisme.* Paris: Nagel, 1970, p. 78.
20 p. 47 in [19].
21 Daniels, N. Reflective equilibrium and Archimedian points. *Canadian Journal of Philosophy*, 1980; 10: 83–103. In this paper Daniels explains the concept of a reflective equilibrium from a *deontological* point of view. However, the English *utilitarian* ethicist R.M. Hare has also stressed that we must aim at a multilevel ethical system comprising intuitions, principles and background theories (R.M. Hare. *Moral thinking. Its Levels, Method and Point.* Oxford: Clarendon Press, 1984, p. 40).

CHAPTER 13
THE ETHICAL DIMENSION OF MEDICAL DECISIONS

*T*extbooks on medical ethics usually devote much space to such controversial topics as euthanasia, death criteria and the abortion problem, but in this brief presentation we have chosen to avoid these difficult problems, and instead we shall discuss the general aspects of ethical reasoning both in clinical practice and in clinical research.

Problems on a ward round

The first patient to be discussed is a middle-aged woman suffering from hyperthyroidism. She is in need of treatment, and the clinician has three options: long-term treatment with anti-thyroid drugs which block hormone synthesis, subtotal thyroidectomy which diminishes the amount of hormone-producing tissue, and administration of a single dose (or a few doses) of radioactive iodine. All these treatments are effective in the large majority of patients, but the advantages and the hazards differ. Drug treatment necessitates medical control for a long period of time and in a few patients the drug may cause serious side-effects; thyroidectomy may cure the patient once and for all, but it involves the risk of immediate operative complications (as well as the risk of damage to the recurrent laryngeal nerve and resulting vocal cord paralysis), whereas radioactive treatment in a considerable number of cases leads to myxoedema (hypofunction of the gland) years later.

First of all, the clinician must make up his mind which decision in his opinion will have the best consequences for the patient, and for that purpose he will act according to the principle of *patient-orientated utilitarianism*. The reasoning process which leads to such a decision is frequently very complicated, as the clinician can rarely predict with certainty what will happen in the individual case. He must choose that decision which on average has the best consequences, and to that end he must consider both the *probability* and the *utility* of all possible events.

Decision theorists have tried to formalize the procedure, and their analysis of 'decision-making under uncertainty' may help to explain the problem.

In principle, the decision-maker must first make a list of all possible outcomes of each decision and, next, he must assess the probability of these outcomes. This is the scientific component of the decision process and, as explained in Chapter 7, the necessary information is often derived from studies on groups of patients. There are, for instance, many articles in the medical literature where clinical investigators have recorded the frequency of a variety of complications of antithyroid therapy.

Then, the decision-maker assesses the value for the patient of each possible outcome. Such evaluations are by necessity inexact, but nevertheless decision theorists expect the decision-maker to indicate the value of each outcome on a utility scale from 0 to 1. The worst possible outcome (sudden death in connection with thyroidectomy) is said to have utility 0, the best possible outcome (complete cure with no therapeutic side-effects) is said to have utility 1, and the utilities of all the other outcomes are fixed somewhere along the scale. For instance, one may decide that the utility of the state of hypothyroidism following treatment with radioactive iodine has utility 0.85.

When this has been done it is easy for the decision theorist to solve the problem; he simply multiplies the probabilities and the utilities, adds up the products for each decision, and then states which decision ensures the highest average utility.

It seems highly unlikely that this procedure will ever be used in practice as no realistic method exists for assessing the utilities in quantitative terms, but the approach is interesting as it correctly reveals the structure of utilitarian thinking. Clinicians may not be able to calculate which is the best decision, but they cannot deny that they must reason along these lines. In this particular case, for instance, the clinician decided that radioactive iodine was best, and he could not have reached that decision in a rational way, except by considering the probability and utility of different outcomes.

The treatment of hyperthyroidism is discussed in all textbooks of medicine, and most doctors would regard it as a purely scientific matter, but the example reveals that even commonplace clinical problems have both a scientific and an ethical component. The assessment of the probabilities definitely belongs to the sphere of natural science, whereas the assessment of the utilities at least in part includes an ethical value judgment. The clinician may, of course, consider which treatment is most effective for normalizing the activity of the thyroid gland and alleviating a particular symptom, but these immediate goals are only *good as means*. The final choice depends on his global assessment of the effect of all the likely desirable and undesirable outcomes on the patient's quality of life, and a good quality of life is *good in itself*. Thus, when we say that the clinician seeks the best consequences for the patients, we mean 'best' in the absolute sense, which is central to ethical considerations.

Philosophers often quote Hume's law which states that one cannot derive an *ought* from an *is*, and this is also applicable to medicine. We may study what there *is* in the world by means of controlled clinical trials and laboratory experiments, but—unless we believe in ethical naturalism (p. 178)—we must agree with Hume that the results of such studies do not tell us how we *ought* to act in a given situation.

Patient-orientated utilitarianism is, like universal act utilitarianism (p. 179), an example of situation ethics, as the decision-maker only considers the consequences of his action in that particular case, but a clinician must also view his decisions in a wider perspective. If, for instance, he is employed in a national health service with a limited budget, he must help to ensure that other patients get a proper share of the limited resources according to their needs. Therefore, he must also consider the *rule utilitarian* approach, which means that he will take into account the general consequences if every clinician makes the same therapeutic decision under similar circumstances. Sometimes clinicians are faced with a choice between several treatments, one of which may be considered marginally better but more expensive than the others, and under such circumstances rule utilitarian considerations may tell him to choose the cheaper treatment. He may conclude that the routine use of the most expensive treatment from the point of view of all patients would do more harm than good by draining the limited resources. In the case of the thyrotoxic patient this dilemma did not arise as the treatment with radioactive iodine is both effective and economic, but it is an important problem in modern hospital practice in general.

We have yet to discuss the deontological considerations. So far, it has been taken for granted that the clinician made the decision on the patient's behalf and we have completely ignored the patient's autonomy. There can be little doubt that paternalistic medicine is still thriving, but in many countries, including the Scandinavian ones and Great Britain, an increasing number of patients regard their doctor as an adviser rather than a guardian and they expect to take an active part in the decision-making process. In this particular case, it may be argued that the only one who can really assess the advantages and disadvantages of the different possible outcomes is the patient herself, and that she must make the choice. If, for instance, she was very fond of singing, she might refuse both thyroidectomy (which may cause vocal cord paralysis) and treatment with radioactive iodine (which may cause hoarseness due to myxoedema). One may conclude that, as an autonomous person, she has the right to choose what she considers best for herself.

This case illustrates that a clinician always has at least three duties: the duty to do what is best for the patient, the duty to consider the interests of society and the duty to respect the patient's autonomy, and it remains to discuss the sequence of the priority of these obligations.

Before we try to tackle that problem, we shall consider another case which presented a different kind of problem. The patient was a middle-aged man who was believed to have a benign stomach ulcer. He was subjected to a gastric resection (removal of part of the stomach), and the histological examination of the resected part unexpectedly revealed the presence of cancer cells. It could not be excluded that the cancer would recur, but no further treatment was considered possible. After the operation, the surgeon had to decide whether he ought to disclose the true diagnosis to the patient. This

The Ethical Dimension of Medical Decisions 191

problem is obviously an ethical one, and the line of reasoning is very much the same as in the previous example. First, the clinician reasoned according to the patient-orientated approach and considered the consequences in this concrete situation of telling or withholding the truth. He felt that there was a good chance that the patient had been cured, and in that case disclosing the true diagnosis would only cause a lot of unnecessary worry. If the cancer recurred, it might be necessary to tell the truth later, but why not let the patient live happily as long as possible? At this stage the doctor also searched his own mind critically to be sure that he was really trying to do the best for the patient. He must take care that he was not in fact thinking of himself (according to the egoistic approach), wishing to avoid an embarrassing conversation.

Next, he viewed this concrete situation in a broader perspective, and, in accordance with a rule utilitarian approach, he considered the consequences of all doctors deciding to withhold the truth under similar circumstances. It would have the effect that a cancer diagnosis would only be disclosed in incurable cases and the population would be misled into believing that cancer is always a fatal disease. In addition, it would inevitably become common knowledge that doctors sometimes lie, and that would cause much unnecessary worry among patients with benign diseases who would not feel reassured when their doctor truthfully denied that the diagnosis was malignant. Until recently, this has been the situation in Denmark and possibly many other countries.

Finally, the clinician must not ignore his patient's rights as an autonomous person. He may sincerely believe that the patient will live more happily in ignorance, but it is by no means certain that the patient wishes to live in a fool's paradise. It may be argued that it is beyond the doctor's competence to conceal the diagnosis and prognosis, and that it is the right of any individual, regardless of consequences, to be told the truth.

In this case the doctor chose to tell the patient in a light tone of voice that it was a good thing that he had been treated surgically, as the examination under the microscope had revealed malignant changes which might have developed into an inoperable growth. The doctor did not tell the patient that the cancer might recur and the patient did not ask. We shall leave it to the reader to decide whether the doctor chose the right level of information.

Before we attempt to analyse the problems which are illustrated by these two case histories, we must consider in some detail the concepts of autonomy and paternalism.

Autonomy and paternalism

Both clinical examples demonstrate the conflict in clinical medicine between utilitarian and deontological thinking, which results from the fact that clinicians must consider the consequences of their actions and at the same time take into account the autonomy of their patients. In the summary which concluded the previous chapter, we wrote that, according to our view, utilitarian considerations must usually give way to those considerations which concern the autonomy of the individual, and we shall now attempt to clarify that vague statement.

The notion of autonomy is ambiguous as it means different things to different philosophers. In Kantian deontological ethics and hermeneutic philosophy, autonomy is regarded as a constituent property of a person. The autonomous person reasons, chooses his own norms and values, plans ahead, makes decisions and acts freely in accordance with these decisions. Philosophers, like Kant and Kierkegaard, may not stress the same elements of this totality of ideas, but they agree that the notion of autonomy is associated with that of the freedom of the individual.

A utilitarian philosopher, like John Stuart Mill, is also devoted to the freedom of individuals, although he is more concerned with the freedom of action than the freedom of the will, and he reconciles this view with his utilitarian position by maintaining that the promotion of autonomy in the long run maximizes the benefits to everybody concerned:

> I regard utility as the ultimate appeal on all ethical questions; but it must be utility in the largest sense, grounded on the permanent interests of a man as a progressive being. Those interests, I contend, authorise the subjection of individual spontaneity to external control, only in respect to those actions of each, which concern the interests of other people [1].

The difference between the views of Kant and Mill may, from a practical point of view, seem very subtle, as both of them stress the importance of the principle of autonomy, but the fundamental utilitarian idea that individual autonomy must be pursued because it is beneficial, just as we pursue other things which are also beneficial, leaves the door ajar to mental utilitarian calculations which balance the degree of freedom against other desirable goals. The Kantian view, that to violate somebody's autonomy is to violate his humanity and to treat him as a thing, is a much stronger and more uncompromising position.

Those who accept the Kantian point of view must oppose utilitarian reasoning when it serves to condone the *principle of paternalism,* i.e. the principle that we are permitted to act on behalf of other people, if we believe that it serves their interests best. However, this view does not imply that paternalism, in the widest sense of the word, must always be condemned, and in order to explain this important point it will be helpful to distinguish between three types: *genuine paternalism, solicited paternalism* and *unsolicited paternalism.*

Genuine paternalism is well illustrated by the father who imposes his will on his small child 'because daddy knows best'. In this situation, paternalistic behaviour will be approved by most people, as it is assumed that the child, because of its immaturity, cannot be regarded as a fully autonomous person, and the medical implications are clear cut. Doctors have among their patients those who are unconscious, delirious because of a high temperature, or severely mentally handicapped, and in all such cases of greatly diminished autonomy, there is no doubt that paternalistic behaviour is needed.

Rawls's defence of genuine paternalism under such circumstances is particularly interesting, as it shows that his *social contract theory* can be applied to medical problems. He writes:

> The problem of paternalism deserves some discussion here, since it ... concerns a lesser freedom. In the original position* the parties assume that in society they are rational and able to manage their own affairs.... But ... they will want to insure themselves against the possibility that their powers are undeveloped and they cannot rationally advance their interests, as in the case of children; or that through some

---
*i.e. under the veil of ignorance (see p. 182).

misfortune or accident they are unable to make decisions for good....

For these cases the parties adopt principles stipulating when others are authorized to act in their behalf and to override their present wishes if necessary ... [2].

Rawls adds that, if possible, paternalistic decisions are to be guided by the individual's own settled preferences: 'We must be able to argue that with the development of the recovery of his rational powers the individual in question will accept our decision on his behalf and agree with us that we did the best thing for him'.

Solicited paternalism is also morally acceptable, as it is implied that the involved person has given his explicit or implicit consent. As an example, one of the authors of this book once visited a small inn in Bosnia, where the menu was hand-written in cyrillic letters and where the inn-keeper only spoke Serbocroatian. The Danish guest remained at the table in spite of the communication gap, and the inn-keeper correctly interpreted this behaviour as a request to act on the guest's behalf and served a delicious meal.

Similar situations frequently occur in medical practice, as many patients feel as lost, when they are admitted to a modern hospital, as the guest in the Bosnian inn, and most of us will agree that it is the patient's right to trust the doctor and to follow his advice. Usually, but not always, the seriously ill patient, who knows nothing about medicine, does not want a long lecture on the advantages and disadvantages of different therapeutic options, but simply expects his doctor to do what in the expert's opinion has to be done.

The only type of paternalism which creates serious ethical problems is the *unsolicited* one. From the Kantian point of view, it is *always* morally wrong to disregard the autonomy of a patient; however, it is not permissible to cut short this discussion with such an uncompromising statement. Many clinicians will, in principle, accept the Kantian concept of a person, but, if they are honest with themselves, they will also have to admit that, under certain circumstances, their intuition tells them that it is best to behave in a paternalistic manner. As explained in the last chapter, it is not sufficient to deduce a moral action principle from a background theory, like the Kantian theory of man; we must aspire to a wide reflective equilibrium which includes intuitive moral judgments as well as background theories and moral principles.

The Ethical Dimension of Medical Decisions

In the second of the two clinical examples, the clinician did not tell the patient the full truth. He mentioned malignant changes, but did not say clearly that the patient already had a cancer and that it could not be excluded that the cancer would recur either in the stomach or, if it had already spread, in some other organ. He felt intuitively that he had chosen the right level of information, but there can be no doubt that his behaviour was paternalistic.

This doctor's behaviour may, of course, be defended on utilitarian grounds by claiming that autonomy is just one kind of good which has to be balanced against other kinds of good, as, for instance, peace of mind. But, if we do not accept that argument, the defence must rest on the idea of an unwritten social contract between doctors and patients. We have already quoted Rawls's arguments in favour of genuine paternalism and, by taking his argument a bit further, it may be suggested that rational people who are planning a society under 'a veil of ignorance' with regards to their future health, would authorize doctors, within certain limits, to withhold information about future events that cannot be avoided, if the doctor believes that such information might ruin their lives. The suggestion is, of course, dangerous as it may be interpreted as a *carte blanche* to those doctors who are inclined to act on their patients' behalf, but it is difficult to deny that there are cases, where most people would feel that it would be unnecessarily cruel to tell the full truth. Few people, we believe, would disapprove of the doctor who did not tell an elderly patient that the routine chest X-ray had revealed an intractable lung cancer which caused no symptoms at all. In such a case it may be argued that the paternalism was not unsolicited and unacceptable, but solicited according to the generally accepted moral norms of society. The doctor did not withhold the truth just because he felt that it was the best decision, but because he had to act in that way as the administrator of a social contract.

The difficulty consists in drawing the line between unsolicited and solicited paternalism, and there is a great need for public debate and descriptive ethical studies which may show what people expect when, for instance, they are admitted to hospital. This is the only way to establish those generally accepted norms which are needed to guide medical practitioners. At present, patients who are admitted to hospital do not know much about the way in which doctors reason, and doctors have to rely almost exclusively on their intuition.

It may be added in this context that it is more than likely that both patients' expectations and doctors' behaviour differ greatly from country to country, so that the efforts to bring all these problems out into the open must take place on a national as well as an international level.

It was stated that genuine paternalism is both necessary and morally permissible, but unfortunately it is also extremely difficult to draw the line between genuine and unsolicited paternalism. Most patients who appear in the consultation room of a general practitioner may be considered autonomous by any standard, but a doctor who receives emergency cases at a hospital will encounter not only a few patients who are clearly incapable of making decisions on their own behalf, but also numerous other patients who, perhaps for a few hours or a few days, require that the doctor acts paternalistically. M. S. Komrad probably goes too far when he asserts that 'all illness represents a state of diminished autonomy' which implies that diminished autonomy is a constituent feature of illness, but he is right when he stresses that the therapeutic relationship between doctor and patient is a dynamic process [3]. We often talk about autonomy as if it was either permanently present or absent, but it is frequently temporarily reduced. The patient who is admitted with strong praecordial pain may be so frightened that he can make no rational decisions, but a few hours later he may be completely relaxed; and the febrile patient with a pneumonia may behave quite irrationally, but when the temperature falls he may again be completely normal. In such cases the doctor will take it in his stride that he sometimes has to give the necessary treatment under mild or even strong protests from the patient. Komrad describes the doctor–patient relationship like this: 'It is a journey from limited paternalism to maximal autonomy which is its *telos*, or ultimate purpose. As the patient's capacity for autonomy increases, so the physician's paternalism which nurtures that autonomy decreases' [3].

The danger is, of course, that the doctor oversteps the borderline between temporary, supportive paternalism of the genuine kind and unacceptable unsolicited paternalism, and the best test is probably the one which was suggested by Rawls: afterwards the patient must 'agree with us that we did the best thing for him'.

It is also necessary to appeal to a social contract theory when a clinician who is employed in a national health service feels that he has to take into account his duty towards society. Rawls's theory implies that people, in order to further their own interests as much as possible, must establish social institutions for their mutual benefit, and it may well be argued that people planning a just society, under a veil of ignorance, would choose to organize a public health service in order to ensure that they would never be deprived of necessary medical treatment. However, if they did that, they would also have to realize that the budget of that health service could not be unlimited, and it would therefore be part of the social contract that those who were delegated the responsibility for the service—in particular the doctors—would have to ascertain that everybody got a fair share according to their needs. This line of reasoning is in perfect harmony with Rawls's idea of distributive justice, and it is not unreasonable to claim that people who live in a democratic country with a public health service have in fact accepted such a contract, and that they are, therefore, morally obliged to permit their doctor to consider the common interest.

The situation is very different in countries where the economy of the health service is seen as part of the market economy in general. However, we shall not enter into a discussion on that topic which borders on political philosophy, but merely point out that this is a good illustration of the fact that the ethics of clinical practice cannot be viewed in isolation. It must accord with the norms and values of society, and those norms and values also determine the organization of social institutions.

The ultimate decision

The last clinical problem to be discussed concerns the importance of assessing a patient's future quality of life, and once again we shall use a clinical example to illustrate the dilemma.

An eighty-year-old man had suffered a stroke which had caused hemiparesis and severe aphasia. He was waiting for transfer to a nursing home, and for several months the condition had been completely stationary. The patient recognized his relatives but did not seem to understand them when they talked to him. When they left the room he seemed distressed and often tried to climb out of bed. One night, this patient developed a septic shock which was caused by a urinary infection, and the young doctor on duty treated this condition successfully with antibiotics, plasma infusion, and other intensive therapeutic measures. We shall presume that the patient would have died if he had not been treated.

Afterwards, the medical staff discussed this case and everybody agreed that in this particular situation it would have been better to let the patient die. The patient had been healthy until he suffered the stroke and there was no longer any hope that he would recover. We can wish no more for ourselves, for those we love, and for our patients, than a long life in good health which is terminated by a brief period of illness.

This conclusion may also be justified by rule utilitarian arguments. If all doctors treat such patients actively, they cause a lot of unnecessary suffering, not only to the patients and their relatives, but also to other elderly people who are afraid of not being allowed to die 'a natural death' if they are admitted to hospital. In Denmark, some people have gone so far as to sign a document which states that they do not wish to be treated actively if there is no chance of a reasonable quality of life.

The deontological aspects of this case are more complex. Everybody will agree that, in the vast majority of cases, it is the professional duty of doctors, whenever possible, to preserve life, and the exceptions to this rule are so rare that it is not surprising that it is sometimes regarded as absolute. Probably, the young doctor did not disagree with the utilitarian arguments, but he made that decision which he believed was intrinsically right, regardless of consequences.

However, it may be argued that doctors' duty to preserve life is not absolute. Death is the inevitable and natural end to all human lives, and one may hold that it is only their duty to preserve life of a certain quality. The value of human life depends on our capacity for self-reflective evaluation and action, and, if this capacity is irrevocably and severely reduced in an eighty-year-old man, abstention from active treatment may be morally required. Cynthia Cohen, who has argued along these lines, writes:

> ... 'Quality of life' considerations are grounded in the recognition that in some tragic instances the lives of valuable human beings can regress to a state in which they bear no reasonable promise of reflecting their self-chosen values. If we

The Ethical Dimension of Medical Decisions   199

insist that such persons must be given intensive medical treatment, we are violating our very belief in the immense value of human beings as reflective deliberators with the capacity to direct their lives according to their conception of well-being [4].

Doctors who accept this point of view will have to conclude, as Cynthia Cohen does, that 'There is as much onus on us to determine that life-saving treatment is required in a particular situation as there is to determine that it is not'.

The problems which are illustrated by the three patients we have discussed in this chapter are so common that they are encountered every day at a modern hospital. Nevertheless, medical students and junior doctors are rarely taught to analyse such problems systematically, and they only learn to act according to the norms of the medical profession, to the extent that such norms exist, by imitating the decisions of their seniors. Of course, as pointed out already, no philosopher can ever solve an ethical dilemma, but we suggest that some knowledge of moral philosophy and systematic analysis of ethical problems may help to ensure that the clinical decision-maker does not overlook important aspects of his problem and that he acts consistently in similar cases.

Ethics and clinical research

The ethics of clinical research is a huge and extremely complex topic, and in this brief presentation of ethical quandaries in medicine we shall confine ourselves to the ethics of the controlled therapeutic trial (p. 44). We shall not go into details but draw a sketch of the structure of the ethical analysis which is required when a clinician wishes to engage himself in that type of research.

Typically, a clinician wishes to compare the effect of two drugs, the one in current use and a new one which may or may not be more effective. He will want to ensure that the results are as reliable as at all possible, and, therefore, he will have to allocate a number of patients with a particular disease at random to the two treatments, and if it is possible, he will take care that the trial is double-blind (i.e. that neither patient nor clinician knows which of the two treatments is given during the trial). The ethical implications of such a trial must be viewed from at least three different angles.

Firstly, the clinician reasons along *universal utilitarian* lines and considers the benefits of the trial for everybody concerned. The primary aim of controlled therapeutic trials—or any other kind of clinical research—is not to benefit those patients who enter the trial, but to benefit future patients with the same disease, and often it may be taken for granted that those benefits will be considerable. The reports of such trials are usually published in international journals, and, consequently, the results may help to ensure that a large number of patients in different countries may henceforth be treated more effectively.

Secondly, the clinician must remember that a research project of this kind in no way relieves him of his duty to do the best for his patients. Therefore, he must also consider the *patient-orientated utilitarian* approach; he must take into account the consequences for those patients who enter the trial, and that poses a difficult problem as he cannot know in advance what the trial will show. He must, of course, make sure that the new drug has been thoroughly tested in the laboratory by means of animal experiments and in preliminary studies on healthy volunteers, and he must refrain from doing the trial if these tests suggest that the patients who receive the new drug are placed at a disadvantage, but he can never be quite sure that the drug has the envisaged effect and that it does not produce unexpected side-effects.

In the Declaration of Helsinki, which was adopted by the World Medical Association in 1964 and revised in 1975 [5], it is stated that 'In any medical study, every patient—including those of a control group, if any—should be assured of the best proven diagnostic and therapeutic method'. If this clause is taken literally, it forbids trials of this nature, as the treatment to be tested does not qualify as 'the best proven therapeutic method', but usually the clause is only taken to mean that patients may not be given a treatment which is known to be inferior.

Thirdly, the clinician must consider the autonomy of his patients, and in clinical research it is particularly important that he does not approach this problem as a utilitarian. He must not regard autonomy as one kind of good which can be balanced against other kinds of good, such as better treatment results in future patients. Instead, he must respect the patients' autonomy unconditionally in accordance with Kantian ethics.

The Ethical Dimension of Medical Decisions

In former days, this deontological consideration was often overlooked as doctors performed controlled trials without informing their patients, but the situation changed after the introduction of the Helsinki Declaration. According to this declaration, it is the doctor's duty to ensure that all patients are

> ... adequately informed of the aim, methods, anticipated benefits and potential hazards of the study and the discomforts it may entail. He or she should be informed that he or she is at liberty to abstain from participation in the study and that he or she is free to withdraw his or her consent to participate at any time. The doctor should then obtain the subject's freely-given informed consent, preferably in writing.

Much has been written on the topic of informed consent, and one of the problems which frequently arises, at least in Denmark, is that the patient wishes to leave the decision to the doctor. The patient receives written information about the trial and then asks the doctor what he thinks. In those cases we usually admit the patient to the trial as we believe that it is the patient's right to delegate responsibility to the doctor. The patient's autonomy is not being violated.

Many controlled trials present no serious ethical problems, but sometimes the utilitarian and deontological considerations collide. For instance, doctors may feel that it is very important for the sake of future patients to do a comparative trial of two treatments, but at the same time they may feel that it is not desirable or possible to obtain the informed consent of the patients who enter the trial. They may, for instance, argue that it would be cruel in cases of malignant diseases with a poor prognosis to tell the patients everything about the inefficiency of the current treatment, and they may hold that it is simply not possible to explain the principles of a trial to severely ill patients who have just been admitted as emergencies.

The Helsinki Declaration contains a much disputed clause which covers these exceptional cases: 'If the doctor considers it essential not to obtain informed consent, the specific reasons for this proposal should be stated in the experimental protocol for transmission to the independent committee'.

According to the Helsinki Declaration, all research projects involving human subjects must be approved by an independent ethical committee, and, according to this clause, it is within the power of that committee to relieve the doctor of his duty to obtain informed consent.

The dilemma is obvious. Intuitively, one may feel that this clause offers a solution to an otherwise insoluble problem, but in principle it makes no difference at all whether the autonomy of a patient is violated by the doctor or by an independent ethical committee. However, once again it may be possible to defend the disregard of the patient's autonomy by resorting to *social contract theory*. It may be argued that most people will agree that it is important that medical science progresses, especially in the treatment of serious diseases, and that, consequently, it is in the common interest to permit controlled trials even when, for some reason or other, it is impossible or undesirable to obtain the consent of each patient. It may also be argued that the decision in such exceptional cases must not be left to the doctor alone, as he might not be completely unbiased, but that it must be endorsed by an independent body which includes both doctors and laymen. At present, however, only a small minority of the population in any country have ever heard about this problem, and under those circumstances it is dangerous to postulate the existence of an unwritten social contract. Also, in this case there is a need for much more public debate and for descriptive studies which record the attitudes in the general population.

The Helsinki Declaration is an example of an international code which is relatively detailed and which has had tremendous beneficial effects, at least in Europe and North America. However, the discussion also shows that it is difficult, even in a limited field, to reach a reflective equilibrium, and the exact guidelines for medical research must be worked out on a national and not on an international level.

Notes and references

1 Mill, J.S. *On Liberty*. Originally published 1859. In: Warnock, M. (ed.) *Utilitarianism*. London: Fontana Collins, 1962, p. 136.
2 Rawls, J. *A Theory of Justice*. Oxford: Oxford University Press, 1971, pp. 248–9.
3 Komrad, M.S. A defense of medical paternalism: maximizing patients' autonomy. *Journal of Medical Ethics*, 1983; 9: 38–44.
4 Cohen, C.B. 'Quality of life' and the analogy with the Nazis. *Journal of Medicine and Philosophy*, 1983; 8: 113–35.
5 Adopted by the 18th World Medical Assembly, Helsinki, Finland, 1964, and revised by the 29th World Medical Assembly, Tokyo, Japan, 1975.

CHAPTER 14
THE MIND AND THE BODY

*I*t is one of the main themes of this book that sick people are not just biological organisms with 'a mechanical fault', but human beings who think, act, hope and suffer. To illustrate this point we presented Kierkegaard's concept of man as an introduction to hermeneutic philosophy, and we discussed Kant's view in the chapters on medical ethics. But we have not yet considered in any detail in which way those states and processes which in medical terminology are called somatic are connected with those which are called mental. We have not considered the relationship between body and mind.

This is a philosophical problem which has intrigued the greatest of thinkers, but it is also important from a medical point of view. Clinicians use their biological knowledge to alleviate their patients' suffering, they classify diseases as mental, somatic or even psychosomatic, and they recognize that they must respect their patients' dignity and autonomy. Medical activity encompasses both the bodily and the mental spheres, and a philosophy of medicine which ignores the relationship between the two is hopelessly incomplete.

Let it be said from the beginning that we are dealing with a philosophical issue which has not yet been settled in a satisfactory way, but we believe that even a limited knowledge of the arguments for and against different mind–body theories may enable the clinician to see the problems of medical research and clinical practice in a wider perspective. The fundamental dilemma was well stated by Immanuel Kant in his *Critique of Pure Reason* in which he explains the difference between causality in nature and human

freedom:
> When we are dealing with what happens there are only two kinds of causality conceivable by us; the causality is either according to *nature* or arises from *freedom*. The former is the connection in the sensible world of one state with a preceding state on which it follows according to a rule.... By freedom, on the other hand, in its cosmological meaning, I mean the power of beginning a state *spontaneously*. Such causality will not, therefore, itself stand under another cause determining it in time, as required by the law of nature [1].

The question is, whether human freedom is an illusion, and Kant formulates this problem by means of an antinomy, i.e. a thesis and an antithesis, both of which can be defended and criticized [2].

According to Kant's thesis, *human beings are free and their mental activities are not caused in the same way as natural phenomena*. This assertion accords well with the subjective experience of all of us that we are free to deliberate about things, to draw our own conclusions from our deliberations and to decide for ourselves what to do in particular situations. Mental processes are not, as physiological processes, subject to the causality of nature, or, as Richard Rorty puts it, 'To suggest that the mind is the brain is to suggest that we secrete theorems and symphonies as our spleens secrete dark humors' [3].

However, in our daily lives we also assume that everything has a natural cause, and we must also seriously consider Kant's antithesis that '*there is no freedom; everything in the world takes place solely in accordance with laws of nature*'.

Gilbert Ryle, a modern philosopher who accepts the antithesis, denounces what he calls 'the dogma of the ghost in the machine' and gives the following scathing description of his opponents' point of view:

> Though the human body is an engine, it is not quite an ordinary engine, since some of its workings are governed by another engine inside it—this interior governor-engine being one of a very special sort. It is invisible, inaudible and it has no size or weight. It cannot be taken to bits and the laws it obeys are not those known to ordinary engines. Nothing is known of how it governs the bodily engine [4].

According to Ryle, such obscure explanations had better be

avoided altogether, but before we are persuaded by his eloquence, we must consider whether we are willing to accept the seemingly inescapable conclusion that our thoughts, our decisions and our behaviour are fully determined by laws of nature. Later, we shall discuss more refined attempts to solve the mind–body problem, but the refinements must not serve to obscure the fundamental issue as it is expressed in Kant's antinomy. It is the very idea of human freedom and human dignity which is at stake.

One of the problems which we face is the elusive character of the word 'mental'. There are many kinds of mental states or events and it is difficult to define clearly what they have in common. Some philosophers have stressed that mental states are intentional, i.e. that they are always directed at something, and there can be no doubt that *intentionality* is a key concept. We do not just hope, we hope for something; we do not just think, we think of something; we always see something, and we decide on something. Especially, continental philosophers, e.g. Heidegger and Brentano, stress this point, but even analytical philosophers agree [5]. Donald Davidson, for instance, writes: 'The distinguished feature of the mental is not that it is private, subjective or immaterial, but that it exhibits what Brentano calls intentionality' [6].

However, Davidson's point of view is debatable. Firstly, some processes that are not usually regarded as mental are also intentional, e.g. the calculation of a P-value by a computer, and, secondly, some states that are clearly mental are not to a convincing degree intentional. Those sensations, like a pain or an itch, which philosophers call 'raw feels', can be localized and described, but they are not directed towards anything in the same way as a hope or a desire. Moods, such as anxiety and depression, also seem to be non-intentional. In Chapter 9 we went so far as to state that anxiety is a constituent property of man, and it was mentioned that it is one of the characteristics of this particular mood that it has no object. Therefore, we do not agree with Davidson that intentionality is the 'distinguished features' of the mental.

Mental states, like the experience of a pain, a sound or a colour, have *phenomenal* properties, which means that they have characteristic qualities which are subjective and private. I know what *I* understand by redness, but I cannot explain in words what this quality is like, and I cannot be sure that others experience redness in the same way. My subjective experience cannot be made objective, but the fact that it exists for me is a proof that I am a conscious being. Other people may ask what it is like to be me, to feel what I feel and to see what I see, but such questions cannot be answered in any objective way. However, by asking the questions they admit that I am a conscious being, as it would make no sense to put the same questions to a motor-car or a computer. The analytical philosopher, Thomas Nagel, expresses this idea in his essay 'What is it like to be a bat?' [7]:

> It is difficult to understand what could be meant by the *objective* character of an experience, apart from that particular point of view from which its subject apprehends it. After all, what would be left of what it was like to be a bat if one removed the viewpoint of the bat?

He also writes:

> But fundamentally an organism has conscious mental states if and only if there is something it is like to *be* that organism—something it is like *for* the organism. We may call this the subjective character of experience. It is not captured by any of the familiar, recently devised reductive analyses of the mental, for all of them are logically compatible with its absence. It is not analyzable in terms of any explanatory system of functional states, or intentional states, since these could be ascribed to robots or automata that behaved like people though they experienced nothing. It is not analyzable in terms of the causal role of experience in relation to typical human behavior—for similar reasons. I do not deny that conscious mental states and events cause behavior, nor that they may be given functional characterizations. I deny only that this kind of thing exhausts their analysis.

Nagel does not go as far as Kierkegaard who asserts that subjective truths are the only ones that matter, but he believes that we must be realists as regards the realm of the subjective, as it is impossible to establish a satisfactory theory of mental phenomena if one does not take into account the subjective qualities of private experience. Kierkegaard expresses the idea as follows: 'The way of objective reflection makes the subject accidental, and therefore transforms existence into something indifferent, something vanishing' (see p. 132). Subjective truths cannot be made objective and attempts to do so make them disappear.

The relation between mind and body was first seen as a central philosophical problem in the 17th century. At that time, the experimental and quantitative methods of natural science gained wide acceptance and it was soon taken for granted that the material part of nature constitutes a closed causal system. Movement was always found to be determined by natural forces, and nature as a whole was regarded as a huge machine, the mechanisms of which must be described mathematically. Nature must be described in quantitative terms, and qualitative experience must be referred to the mind or the soul.

René Descartes (1596–1650) was the first scientist and philosopher to analyse the mind–body problem along these lines. He distinguishes between two separate substances, the corporal one (the body) and the mental one (*res cogitans* = the thinking thing), which are united in man and interact in an extremely intricate way. The basic features of these substances differ:

> Thus, extension in length, breadth and depth constitutes the nature of the corporal substance, and thought constitutes the nature of the mental substance. For everything else which can be attributed to a body presupposes extension and is no more than a feature of this extended thing, just as all the properties which we find in the mental substance are only different forms of thought [8].

A theory of this kind is labelled *dualism*, and the crucial problem which faces all dualists is to explain how two substances of different natures are capable of interaction. Descartes is particularly vague on this point, and in a letter to Princess Elizabeth of Bohemia he only suggests that: 'It is just by means of ordinary life and conversation, by abstaining from meditation and from studying things that exercize the imagination, that one learns to conceive the union of soul and body' [9].

Descartes also suggested that the soul is localized in the pineal body, and this odd idea did little to elucidate the problem.

Later, Baruch de Spinoza (1632–77) opposed Descartes' views and developed a *monistic* theory. He objected to the idea that interaction is possible between body and mind if they are of a different nature, and he arrived at the conclusion that there is only *one* substance (which he calls God or Nature) and that the mental and physical worlds are no more than different aspects or attributes of that substance. The mental and physical aspects are not substantially different, but represent little more than two ways of looking at the same thing. Thoughts are thoughts about certain objects, and objects are objects for certain thoughts. There is no substantial difference between a perception, the perceived object and the perceiver's body, as a perception is regarded as a-state-of-my-body-caused-by-another-body. Unlike Descartes, Spinoza need not worry about the way in which mind and body interact; from his point of view there is no interaction as mental and physical phenomena are seen as two aspects of the same events, but he faces another problem which is equally crucial: his theory is incompatible with the idea of human freedom when this word is used in its ordinary sense. Spinoza fully accepts this consequence of the theory and simply asks us to accept that we are part of nature as a whole and that we must follow its order:

> If we have a clear and distinct understanding of this, that part of our nature which is defined by intelligence, in other words the better part of ourselves, will assuredly acquiesce in what befalls us, and in such acquiescence will endeavour to persist [10].

The conflict between dualism and monism—as well as that between Kant's thesis and antithesis—is as unsettled today as it was then, but progress in the fields of neurophysiology, psychology and philosophy has increased our understanding of the problems, and we shall now turn our attention to some of the modern theories.

Logical behaviourism

The empiricists' solution of the mind–body problem is radical and easy to understand, but perhaps less easy to accept. As explained in Chapter 2, empiricists require that all scientific theory is derived from observed facts and, therefore, the qualitative subjective experiences of the individual are expelled from the realm of science. The foremost exponent of this point of view is the British philosopher Gilbert Ryle (1900–76) who, as mentioned on page 204, denounces the dogma of the ghost in the machine.

Ryle believes that the mind–body problem is a pseudo-problem which is the result of conceptual misunderstandings. It is generally assumed that mental concepts like intelligence, shyness, anger, jealousy, etc., are properties of a person's soul, in much the same way as blueness of the eyes or obesity are properties of a person's body. However, according to Ryle, there is no object which is characterized by being intelligent, as intelligence is no more than a word which signifies certain types of behaviour or dispositions to behave in certain ways. An intelligent person is someone who can solve intellectual problems, e.g. mathematical ones, more quickly than others. Similarly, there is no object which is characterized by being shy, as shyness is just a word which signifies a disposition to blush and to behave in an awkward manner. Ryle stresses that mentalistic terms can be eliminated altogether, as, logically, they are redundant. Ryle's behaviourism represents a radical attempt to cut the Gordian knot, but as a theory it is not convincing. It is true, of course, that there is a strong correlation between subjective experience and behaviour, as illustrated by the fact that we can often observe that a person is happy, shy or in pain, but most people will agree that the behaviourists go too far when they disregard subjective experience and identify, say, pain with pain behaviour. From a behaviourist point of view, it is not possible to distinguish between a person who is in pain and exhibits pain behaviour, and a person who is not in pain but imitates pain behaviour, as the behaviourist ignores the subjective fact that pain hurts and that it is the hurtfulness of the pain which causes the behaviour. As explained on page 113, behaviourist theory leaves no room for the idea that mental states may be causally active.

However, in spite of its shortcomings the behaviourist theory has catalysed much important empirical research in the fields of both animal and human psychology. It has also had some influence on modern psychiatry, and in Chapter 8 we discussed the behaviourist approach to the concept of mental disease.

The causal theory of the mind

The empiricist point of view that scientific theories must be based on observed facts is highly unsatisfactory when we are dealing with mental phenomena, and the behaviourist approach was doomed to failure. Even modern scientific theories which only concern the physical world make use of theoretical entities, such as energy, magnetic fields and elementary particles, that are not directly observable, and from a *realist* point of view it makes just as much sense to accept the existence of conscious and unconscious mental states and processes, if these concepts form part of a consistent theory of the workings of the mind.

The most reasonable starting-point is our actual understanding of the way in which mental phenomena, like feelings, moods and wishes, determine our actions. We must maintain that feelings play *a causal role* and that it is the feeling of pain which makes us cry, the feeling of hunger which makes us eat and the feeling of fear which makes us flee. Similarly, we must maintain that moods are not just types of behaviour, but inner states which *cause* modifications of our behaviour. Anxiety, for instance, is not the same as anxiety behaviour, but a state of mind which affects the manner in which a person conducts himself. But this description of the workings of the mind is not exhaustive. Mental phenomena do not only cause or modify our immediate actions; they may also cause other mental phenomena, and they can be stored in the mind with the result that they determine our behaviour at a much later state. The experience of a bodily assault on a dark night may cause feelings of fear or anger which determine the immediate actions, but the experienced course of events and the resulting feelings will be remembered, and the stored mental phenomena may have the effect that the person in future will be more reluctant to go for a walk after sunset. Our behaviour is determined by a complex network of interacting mental states and processes.

Mental phenomena are often concealed inner causes of our actions, but those mental states and events which have *phenomenal* properties (see p. 205) are directly accessible by introspection. Feelings, like pain, itching, fear, jealousy or remorse, are not purely theoretical, but can be experienced directly, and it is absurd to exclude such phenomena from a theory of the workings of the mind.

It is important to realize that the causal theory of mind, as it has been presented here, is non-committal as regards the conflict between monism and dualism. We have only asserted that mental states play a causal role in our patterns of action and that they cannot be reduced to behaviour (or dispositions to behave). The true nature of mental phenomena remains to be settled, and we shall now consider three theories (the identity theory, functionalism and a modern version of dualism) which provide very different answers to that problem. All three theories are compatible with the causal theory of the mind.

The identity theory

The identity theory (which is also called physicalistic monism or central-state materialism) is as radical as behaviourism. It is simply assumed that mental states and processes are *identical with* neurophysiological states and processes in the central nervous system. From the point of view of the medical scientist, it is tempting to accept this theory, as it is well established that a close association exists between brain function and the workings of the mind, and to some extent the identity theory may be regarded as the philosophical basis of the biological concept of mental disease, which was discussed in Chapter 8. The theory, however, presents serious problems, some of which were mentioned at the beginning of this chapter.

Firstly, those who accept the identity theory must also accept Kant's antithesis. It is reasonable to assume that nature is a closed causal system and that all phenomena in nature, including neurophysiological processes, are fully determined by antecedent states and events. Therefore, the identity theory involves the point of view that our actions are always predetermined and that human autonomy is an illusion. Of course, it is possible to retain the idea of human freedom, if freedom is redefined in such a way that we are regarded as 'free agents' when our predetermined actions are not impeded by external causes, but it still seems difficult to reconcile concepts like moral responsibility and guilt with this deterministic view of man.

Secondly, the identity theory (like behaviourism) is vulnerable to Nagel's criticism that it does not capture the notion of subjective experience. A toothache is identified with a certain state of the brain, but that idea does not account for the hurtfulness of *my* toothache, and it does not exclude the possibility that other people, whose brains are in the same state, experience their toothache in a different way. A theory which reduces mental phenomena to neurophysiology does not capture a problem of this kind, as the reduction has the effect that the subjective character of the sensation is ignored. The identity theory is a good illustration of

Kierkegaard's statement that subjective truths cannot be made objective, as attempts to do so make them vanish.

Thirdly, the claim of an identity between mental and neurophysiological states presents logical problems. Leibnitz's law states that identical objects have identical properties, and, if the identity theory is true, mental states and those neurophysiological states with which they are identified must fulfil this requirement. That, however, does not seem to be the case. Imagine that I close my eyes and that I visualize to myself the rectangular yellow piece of paper on which I am writing. If my table is well lit, I may even have an after-image of this piece of paper. In that case I am in a mental state which is characterized by the properties 'yellow' and 'rectangular'. According to the identity theory, it is then to be expected that the state of my brain is also characterized by 'yellowness' and 'a rectangular shape', and obviously this assumption is ridiculous. Attempts have been made to counter this simple argument, but the solutions are not entirely convincing. Recently, the American philosopher Saul Kripke has produced much stronger logical arguments against the identity claim [11], but a discussion of his refutation of the identity theory is beyond the scope of this book.

In order to avoid such problems, it has been postulated that some mental states, apart from being neurophysiological states, have the additional characteristic that they are experienced in a certain manner. This theory, which is called *epiphenomenalism*, is a kind of dualism, as it is admitted that some mental states have both material and non-material properties, but it is maintained that only neurophysiological processes play a causal role. The non-material phenomena—the qualitative contents of our subjective experience—are only regarded as by-products (epiphenomena) of the workings of the brain, just like 'smoke from a chimney' or 'a shadow on the wall'. This theory has the advantage over the identity theory that it takes into account subjective experience, but but it does not tell us anything about the nature of the epiphenomena or the way in which they are produced.

Functionalism

In recent years, a much more sophisticated mind–body theory has been developed by, among others, Hilary Putnam [12].

According to this theory, the central nervous system has physical properties, but it also has other properties which are not of a physical nature, i.e. which can be specified and defined without reference to the anatomy and physiology of the brain. This idea, which at first may be difficult to grasp, is well illustrated by the properties of a computer. The computer is a machine with physical properties, as it is composed of a multitude of electrical circuits, but it also has functional properties. It may, for instance, be programmed to execute a chi-square test, and this program can be described in every detail in mathematical and logical terms without reference to the physical structure of the computer. Other computers which are constructed in a completely different way can be programmed to execute exactly the same test. The chi-square program of course requires some sort of physical realization, but this realization may take many forms: the program may simply be written on a piece of paper, it may have been fed into a computer or it may be stored somewhere in a statistician's brain. It may be a non-physical property of a piece of paper, a computer or a human brain.

The example illustrates the functionalist's approach to the mind–body problem. Mental states cannot be reduced to physical ones, and their relation to the brain is analogous to the relation between computer 'software' and computer 'hardware'. Consider, for instance, the feeling of jealousy. This mental state can be realized in different people, it can to some extent be described independently of any particular realization, and it is causally operative. The computer which is fed with the chi-square program produces chi-square values and the jealous person produces a characteristic kind of behaviour. However, jealousy need not be permanent; it may be replaced by another mental state—another program—and then the behavioural 'output' will change.

Functionalism is the most advanced mind–body theory which has been developed within the empiricist tradition. It is much more acceptable than earlier monistic theories, as for instance behaviourism and the identity theory, and it has provided a valuable conceptual framework for empirical research in the cognitive sciences, e.g. cognitive psychology, psycholinguistics, perception theory, cybernetics and artificial intelligence. It has even proved possible to reinterpret earlier theories from a functionalistic point of view. Freudian psychology, for instance, may be regarded as a premature functionalistic theory, in which the id, ego and superego may be regarded as functional entities which play a role in the development of different mental states [13].

Functionalism is also superior to behaviourism and the identity theory in so far as it captures the *intentional* character of at least some mental states. It was mentioned on page 205 that a mental state, like hoping, is intentional, as we do not just hope, but hope for something, and the same may be said of a computer program; the chi-square program does not just calculate, it calculates a chi-square value. However, like the monistic theories, it still does not capture the notion of subjective qualitative experience. Once again we may imagine a number of people with toothache. They are in the same functional state—the same program is running in their brains—but that idea does not encompass the hurtfulness of the pain and the possibility that these people experience their pain differently. The analogy between mental states and computer programs is in many respects a valuable one, but it ignores the subjective dimension of mental phenomena. Computers do not experience anything and, as pointed out by Nagel, the analysis of a mental state, like a toothache, is incomplete, if it does not take into account what it is like to have a toothache.

Some functionalists [13] recognize that self-reflection is an essential human characteristic, i.e. they accept the importance of 'the spirit' or 'the self' which constitutes the third element in Kierkegaard's analysis of man (Chapter 9). However, their attempts to give a satisfactory account of the nature of self-reflection within the conceptual framework of functionalism has not been altogether successful.

Interactionistic dualism

At the beginning of this chapter, we briefly presented Descartes' dualistic and Spinoza's monistic mind–body theories, and, on the preceding pages, we have described how most philosophers in this century have followed in Spinoza's footsteps. More and more sophisticated monistic theories have been developed and, to quote Dennett, 'It is widely granted these days that dualism is not a serious view to contend with, but rather a cliff over which to push one's opponents' [14].

However, one prominent philosopher, Karl Popper, does not agree with this view. In their book with the telling title *The Self and its Brain* [15], Karl Popper and the neurophysiologist J. C. Eccles present a modern version of dualism. We shall briefly explain their theory which is part of Popper's three-world philosophy.

World 1 is the material world. It contains objects and structures as diverse as metals, trees, brain cells, chairs and computers, and from the point of view of many natural scientists, it is the only world which exists.

World 2 is the world of conscious experience, which includes perception, thought, feeling, mood, memory and self-awareness. In other words, it is the private world of the mind or the self. Behaviourists and identity theorists deny the existence of this world, but to Popper this denial is 'clearly wrong, even though irrefutable'. He writes in his memoirs:

> That we do experience joy and sadness, hope and fear, not to mention a toothache, and that we do think, in words as well as by means of schemata; that we can read a book with more or less interest and attention—all this seemed to me obviously true, though easily denied; and extremely important, though obviously non-demonstrable. It also seems to me quite obvious that we are embodied selves or minds or souls [16].

World 3 is the world of all cultural products, like languages, works of art and scientific theories. Many World 3 objects are embodied in World 1 objects—scientific theories are printed in books and sculptures are carved in stone—but the objects of World 3 are also themselves real. The contents of books exist—and the scientific theories which are printed in them are true or false—even when nobody reads the books; and the written language of the ancient Egyptians existed, even in those days when nobody could decipher the hieroglyphics.

According to Popper, World 2 (the mind) interacts both with World 1 (the material world) and World 3 (the world of cultural products), whereas World 1 and World 3 do not interact except through the mediation of World 2. Human beings, for instance, perceive the colours of the objects which surround them (World 1 → World 2), they learn to speak and write (World 3 → World 2), they often decide to move objects from one place to another (World 2 → World 1) and, if they are particularly gifted, they produce valuable works of art (World 2 → World 3).

Popper and Eccles have developed a theory which agrees well with the idea of human freedom, but the fundamental problems remain unsolved. They write somewhat vaguely that the conscious mind reads out from, selects from and acts upon the 'liaison areas' of the cerebral hemispheres, but they do not tell us how it is able to do so. They are reintroducing the ghost in the machine, which Ryle so elegantly expelled from philosophy years ago, and lose themselves in vague metaphors. Human beings can 'read', 'select' and 'act' but it makes little sense to bestow these attributes on a mythical entity called mind.

A recapitulation

We agree with Popper that behaviourism as a philosophical thesis was clearly wrong in its denial of the existence of human consciousness. There can be no doubt at all that man is a conscious being and that mental phenomena cannot be analysed satisfactorily in behavioural terms. We must be realists as regards mental states and we must look upon mental states as causes of behaviour. However, the causal theory of the mind is non-committal as regards the true nature—the ontological status—of mental phenomena, and it still remains a problem to what extent such phenomena can be reduced to physical states and processes in the central nervous system. The identity theory has been refuted, as the identity claim does not resist a logical analysis, but the functionalists, who accept the existence of non-material functional states, have captured at least some of the characteristics of mental phenomena. However, their theory does not take into account such notions as conscious perception, self-awareness, self-understanding and human autonomy; it ignores those properties of man which determine his dignity and his ability to make a moral choice. Like other monists, the functionalists are thinking in terms of Kant's antithesis. The inadequacy of monistic theories forces us to reconsider the dualistic alternative, but, as explained above, Popper's and Eccles' theory is equally inadequate.

At present, it is impossible to choose between monism and dualism, and it may be necessary simply to draw the conclusion that we have at our disposal two modes of description which seem mutually irreconcilable. On one hand, we can describe man in biological and behavioural terms, and this naturalistic approach has served to guide empirical science in a number of fields. On the other hand, it is necessary to use mentalistic terms for the description of feelings, moods, hopes and wishes. The medical practitioner has to deal with suffering, anxiety and despair, he must respect his patients' autonomy, and he often faces moral dilemmas. These aspects of medical practice demonstrate that man is a conscious, self-reflecting being, and they imply that the mentalistic and intentional language is as important as the scientific one.

The best methods for studying those phenomena which concern our subjectivity have not yet been sufficiently developed [17], but they must reflect the ideas of Kierkegaard, Heidegger, and other hermeneutic philosophers, which were presented earlier in this book (Chapters 9 and 10). It was concluded then that the analysis of medical problems requires both a scientific and a hermeneutic approach, and the discussion in this chapter of the mind-body problem points in the same direction.

Notes and references

1 Kant, I. *Kritik der reinen Vernunft*. Originally published 1787. English translation by Norman Kemp Smith: *Critique of Pure Reason*, 2nd edn. London: Macmillan, 1933, p. 464 (A532–3).
2 We are referring to Kant's third antinomy, pp. 409ff in [1].
3 Rorty, R. *Philosophy and the Mirror of Nature*. Oxford: Basil Blackwell, 1980, p. 43.
4 Ryle, G. *The Concept of Mind*. Harmondsworth: Penguin Books, 1963, p. 21.
5 Modern analytical philosophers belong to the empiricist tradition. They stress the importance of the analysis of language and logic.
6 Davidson, D. Mental events. In: Block, N. (ed.) *Readings in the Philosophy of Psychology*. London: Methuen, 1980, Vol. 1, p. 109.
7 Nagel, T. What is it like to be a bat? In: Nagel, T. *Mortal Questions*. Cambridge: Cambridge University Press, 1979, pp. 165–79.
8 Descartes, R. *Oeuvres philosophiques*. Originally published 1643–50. Paris: Garnier Frères, 1973, Vol. 3, p. 123.
9 Descartes, R. *Philosophical Writings*. A selection translated and edited by E. Anscombe & P.T. Geach. London: The Open University, 1970, p. 280.
10 Spinoza, B. de. *Ethica*. Originally published 1677. English translation by R. H. M. Elwes. *The Chief Works of Benedict de Spinoza*. New York: Dover, 1955, p. 243.
11 Kripke, S. *Naming and Necessity*. Oxford: Basil Blackwell, 1980.
12 Putnam, H. Mind, language, and reality. *Philosophical Papers*, Vol. 2. Cambridge: Cambridge University Press, 1975.
13 Dennett, D.C. *Brainstorms. Philosophical Essays on Mind and Psychology*. Hassocks: Harvester, 1979.

14 Dennett, D.C. Current issues in the philosophy of mind. *American Philosophical Quarterly*, 1978; **15**: 249–61.
15 Popper, K.R. & Eccles, J.C. *The Self and its Brain*. Berlin: Springer International, 1981.
16 Popper, K. *Unended Quest. An Intellectual Autobiography*. London: Fontana Collins, 1976, p. 187.
17 Grünbaum, A. *The Foundations of Psychoanalysis. A Philosophical Critique*. Berkeley; University of California Press, 1984, p. 21 ff. In this book Grünbaum argues strongly against the 'epistemic primacy' of the patient as claimed by hermeneutic philosophers and psychoanalysts. He holds that psychoanalysis must be governed by the same criteria of validation as the natural sciences.

INDEX OF NAMES

Abel, T. 163
Adler, A. 159, 166
Austin, J. 180

Becker, H.S. 115
Bentham, J. 179
Berkeley, G. 17
Beveridge, W.H. 51–2
Bhaskar, R. 27–8
Bliss, B.P. 177
Boorse, C. 49–51, 53–55
Boyle, R. 16
Brentano, F. 205

Cameron, N. 157
Carnap, R. 19
Cassell, E. 57
Cohen, C. 198–9
Comte, A. 17, 35
Cullen, W. 31, 38

Daniels, N. 184
Darwin, C. 6
Davidson, D. 205
Dennett, D.C. 214
Descartes, R. 207

Eccles, J.C. 215–16
Einstein, A. 6
Engelhardt, H.T. 53
Erikson, E. 160
Eysenck, H.J. 169

Feinstein, A.R. 82
Forster, E.M. 13
Foudraine, J. 105

Freud, A. 159
Freud, S. 157–62, 166–7
Fromm, E. 152

Gadamer, H-G. 123, 142, 146–9, 164
Gavaret, J. 35–9, 44–5

Habermas, J. 142, 149–54, 162
Hacking, I. 27
Hahnemann, S. 31
Hamilton, M. 109–10
Harré, R. 27, 142, 153
Hartmann, H. 160
Harvey, W. 16, 32
Heidegger, M. 123, 125, 129, 133, 164, 205
Hesslow, G. 167
Horney, K. 160
Hume, D. 17, 18, 19, 43, 189

Jaspers, K. 160
Johnsen, S.G. 38–9, 41, 42
Johnson, A.G. 177
Jung, C. 159

Kant, I. 25, 174, 177, 181–2, 192–3, 203–4, 216
Kendell, R.E. 51, 52, 110
Kepler, J. 16
Kierkegaard, S. 123–34, 162, 192, 217
Klein, M. 159
Komrad, M.S. 196
Kraepelin, E. 108
Kräupl-Taylor, F. 54

219

Index

Kripke, S. 212
Krogh-Jensen, P. 83
Kuhn, T.S. 1–7, 11, 12, 102, 118

Laing, R.D. 105–6
Lasègue, E.C. 42
Lesche, C. 162, 165, 169
Linnaeus, C. 34, 75
Locke, J. 17, 25, 26, 33, 74–5, 77–8, 86, 88
Lorenzer, A. 162, 164, 169
Louis, P.C.A. 35, 37

Mach, E. 19
Mackie, J.L. 64, 176
Magee, B. 22
Medawar, P. 22
Mill, J.S. 179, 192
Murphy, E.A. 48

Nagel, T. 206
Newton, I. 16

Pariser, S.F. 117
Pavlov, I. 113
Plato 82
Popper, K.R. 11, 12, 22–4, 26, 161–2, 166–7, 215–16
Praag, H.M. van 106
Putnam, H. 212

Quine, W.V. 80

Rachman, S.J. 169
Rapaport, D. 160
Rawls, J. 182–3, 193–4
Ricoeur, P. 162
Rorty, R. 204
Ross, A. 50, 55, 107
Rousseau, J.-J. 78
Russell, B. 22, 178
Ryle, G. 113, 204, 208–9

Sartre, J.P. 123, 183–4
Sauvages, F. Boissier de 34, 75
Scadding, J.G. 50
Secord, P.F. 142, 153
Skinner, B.F. 113
Smart, J.J.C. 27
Spinoza, B. de 207–8
Sullivan, H.S. 160
Sydenham, T. 33
Szasz, T.S. 105

Watkins, J. 141
Watson, J.B. 113
Weber, M. 141
Wilson, G.T. 169
Winch, P. 142, 143–6, 163
Wittgenstein, L. 4, 144

INDEX OF SUBJECTS AND DEFINITIONS

Page numbers in **bold** print indicate where important words are defined or explained

Act utilitarianism   179
Aetiology   74, 77, 79, 83–4
Analytical hermeneutics   143–6
Angst   **122**, 124–30
Anti-psychiatry   105
Anti-realism   15
Anxiety   109, 117, 121–2, 124–30, 157–8, 162
Autonomy   185, 190, 191, **192**–7, 200–2, 211, 216

Bayesian diagnosis   95–7
Bayes' theorem   96, 97, 102
Behaviourism   113–15, 208–9, 216
Biological concept of disease   46, 111–12, 211
Biological psychiatry   111–12
Biological reductionism   47, 117
Bio-psycho-social disease concept   117, 137, 139, 141

Categorical imperative   174, 181–2
Causality   19, 27, 61–72, 204, 209–11
Causal theory of the mind   209–11, 216
Central-state materialism   211
Clinical syndromes   75, 86–7
Confidence limits   36, 44, 90, 95
Consequentialist ethical theories   179–81
Constituent attributes   **124**–5, 129, 173–4

Critical clinical school   8, 37, 43, 108, 115, 139
Critical theory   149–54

Definition   4
Demarcation criterion   20, 166
Deontology   175, **181**–4, 190, 198
Descriptive ethics   175, 195
Disease classification   73–88, 109
Disease concept   46–9, 105–18
Dualism   207, 214–17

Eclectic view of mental disease   116–18
Effective causal complex   63–4
Egoism   180, 191
Emancipatory interest   151–2
Emotivism   20, **178**
Empathic understanding   58, 162–3
Empiricism   **15**, 16–22, 33–7, 43–5, 62, 71, 94, 109–11, 130–1, 136–43, 154, 166, 178, 208, 213
Epidemiological concept of disease   136
Epiphenomenalism   212
Epistemology   **14**, 27, 143–4
Essentialism   87
Existentialism   123, 184

Falsifiability   22–5, 161, 167
Frequential probabilities   **90**, 93–5
Functionalism   170, 212–14, 216
Fundamental human interests   151

221

Index

Generative theory of causation 19, 62–3, 139–40
Genuine paternalism **193–7**

Helsinki Declaration 8, 200–2
Hermeneutic circle 147
Hermeneutic interest 151–2
Hermeneutics **123**, 125, 130–4, 143–9, 154, 162–6, 169, 192
Holistic view of disease 117, 126, 137
Homeopathy 31
Homeostasis 71
Horizon of understanding 147 ·
Human interests 151
Humean theory of causation 19, 62, 140
Humoral pathology 30–1
Hypothetical imperative 174

Identity theory 211–12, 216
Ideology 150
Induction 20–1, 27, 80
Intentionality 205, 214
Interactionistic dualism 214–17
Inter-subjectivity 19, 146, 163

Laws of nature 19, 27, 36, 204
Logical behaviourism 208–9

Mechanical model 46–49, 111, 136, 178
Meta-ethics **175**, 176–9, 184
Metaphysics 16
Methodological individualism 141
Mind-body theories 128, 203–17
Monism 207–8

Naturalism (ethical) 178
Natural kinds 78, 80
Necessary causal factor 62
Nominalism 77–8, 87
Non-redundant causal factor 63–8, 76
Normality 47–50, 55, 107
Normal science 5, 6, 7, 11
Normative ethics 175
Null hypothesis 100

Objective truth 131–2
Objectivity 19, 206
Ontology 14–16, 27, 54, 111, 115, 216

Paradigm 2, 47, 102, 118
Paternalism **193–7**
Pathogenesis 74, 76, 79, 83–4
Patient-orientated utilitarianism **181**, 188–9, 191, 200
Phenomenal properties 205
Phenomenology 123
Phobia 122
Platonist disease concept 81–8
Positivism 17, 35, 178
Pre-understanding 147–8, 165
Psychoanalysis 152, 157–71
Psychodynamic theories 159
Psychotherapy 159, 169
P-values 99–103

Quality of life 9, 189, 197, 198

Rationalism **15**, 25, 31
Realism **14**, 25–8, 30–3, 37–9, 62–3, 94, 136, 139, 206, 209
Research ethics 199–202
Rule utilitarianism **180**, 189, 191, 198

Scientific revolution 5
Significance tests 99–103
Social contract theory 183, 193, 195, 197, 202
Social psychiatry 115–16
Solicited paternalism **194–7**
Species design 49, 106–7
Speculative realism 30–2
Statistical concept of normality 48
Statistical decision theory 102, 178, 188
Statistical probability concept 90
Subjective probabilities 91–5, 98
Subjective truth 131–2, 165
Succession theory 19, 27, 62, 140
Sufficient causal factor 62

Technical interest 151
Technique 40
Technology 40

Unsolicited paternalism **194–7**
Utilitarianism 175, **179–81**, 183, 192, 198, 200

Verifiability 19, 20, 166
Vienna Circle 17, 143

Wide reflective equilibrium 184–6